Learning from Medical Errors: Legal Issues

Anh Vu T Nguyen
MD, FAAFP

and

Dung A Nguyen
MD, FAAFP

Foreword by David S Starr

Radcliffe Publishing
Oxford • Seattle

Radcliffe Publishing Ltd
18 Marcham Road
Abingdon
Oxon OX14 1AA
United Kingdom

www.radcliffe-oxford.com
Electronic catalogue and worldwide online ordering facility.

British Library Cataloguing in Publication Data
A catalogue record for this book is available from the British Library.

ISBN 1 85775 767 X

Typeset by Ann Buchan (Typesetters), Shepperton, Middlesex, UK
Printed and bound by TJ International Ltd, Padstow, Cornwall, UK

Contents

Foreword

Dr J walked out of the emergency room, tired after a 12-hour day in the front lines of clinical medicine. Waiting for him in the lobby was a process server, a heavily built man in a dark suit, looking for all the world like a detective or insurance salesman. He handed Dr J an envelope, and ignoring the look of stupefaction on the physician's face, quickly turned and walked out through the automatic doors. Another lawsuit had started. Three years later, after countless hearings and depositions, Dr J retired early from clinical medicine, suffering from terminal litigation fatigue.

Today's physician is under pressures that physicians of prior generations would find hard to imagine. The trust that lies at the foundation of the physician–patient relationship has, through unrelenting assault by the forces of government and media, been eroded, and what we are left with is a commercial relationship, devoid of the warmth and confidence that characterized the physician–patient relationship for centuries. Today's physician needs a guide to help him navigate the legal fall-out from this social development, and the authors, Dr Anh Vu and his brother, Dr Dung Nguyen, have provided one, and one that is very well written. In *Learning from Medical Errors: Legal Issues*, the companion book to *Learning from Medical Errors: Clinical Problems,* they deal systematically with the causes and effects of medical errors that have a disturbing tendency to creep into our medical practices unless we take positive steps to prevent them. All of us can benefit from a review of our clinical practices through the eyes of the authors' text, and their work brings a rigor and thoroughness to the analysis that satisfies our sense of professionalism. Their many examples, some of which are drawn from my work in *Cortlandt Forum*, are well chosen and instructive.

I recommend this text to physicians who are seeking a comprehensive text to help them avoid litigation and improve their quality of care.

David S Starr, MD, JD
July 2005

David S Starr, MD, JD practiced law and medicine in Georgetown, Texas for many years. He recently retired from a consulting practice in medicolegal issues, mainly malpractice defense.

List of cases

About the authors

Dr Anh Vu Nguyen was born in Saigon, Vietnam and grew up in Tampa, FL. He attended the University of South Florida as a National Merit Scholar and graduated summa cum laude with a Bachelor of Science in Engineering degree. He then attended the University of South Florida College of Medicine and graduated in 1996. Dr A Nguyen completed his family practice residency at Bayfront Medical Center in Saint Petersburg, FL in 1999 and became board-certified through the American Board of Family Practice. He then moved to Tallahassee, FL. Since then, he has been a full-time emergency physician at Tallahassee Community Hospital (now Capital Regional Medical Center), serving as associate director from 1999–2001. From 1998–2003, Dr A Nguyen also worked part-time as an urgent care provider in Saint Petersburg, FL and in Tallahassee, FL and also as a medical and legal consultant for the Florida Department of Health. In 2003, Dr A Nguyen began serving as a part-time emergency physician at the Bay Pines Veterans Administration Hospital in Saint Petersburg, FL. He obtained board certifications in ambulatory medicine in 2003 through the American Board of Ambulatory Care and in emergency medicine in 2004 through the American Association of Physician Specialists. He has written numerous articles for *Consultant* and *Patient Care* medical journals. Dr Nguyen became a clinical assistant professor at the Florida State University College of Medicine in 2004.

His hobbies include reading, traveling, movies, and the martial arts. He is a second degree black belt from the WTF in Taekwondo and is currently an assistant instructor for the FSU Taekwondo club.

Dr Dung Nguyen is the older brother of Dr A Nguyen and was also born in Saigon, Vietnam. He grew up in Tampa, FL and attended the University of South Florida as a National Merit Scholar and graduated magna cum laude with a Bachelor of Science in Engineering degree. He then attended the University of South Florida College of Medicine and graduated in 1994. Dr D Nguyen completed his family practice residency at Tallahassee Memorial Hospital in Tallahassee, FL in 1997 and became board-certified in family practice. He has been in private practice in Tallahassee since finishing residency. His practice includes both family medicine and urgent care medicine. Dr D Nguyen became board-certified in ambulatory medicine in 2003. From 1999–2001, he served as a medical consultant for the Office of Research and Practice at the University of South Florida. Dr D Nguyen has also been a clinical instructor for the Florida State University College of Medicine since 2002. He has been published in *Patient Care* medical journal.

His hobbies include sports cars, music, traveling, and the martial arts. He is a third degree black belt from the WTF in Taekwondo and is currently an assistant instructor for the FSU Taekwondo club.

Dedications

Our parents, Lan T and Nham T Nguyen, for their tireless devotion to the welfare and education of their children.

Our grandmother, Ca T Nguyen, for the things that she taught us that could not be learned in school.

In appreciation of

We would like to give thanks to Frank J Edwards MD and Steven M Selbst MD. They graciously allowed us to use their cases and gave us encouragement.

We are especially indebted to Jennifer Steimle MD and Shirley Swanson RN for their help in reviewing the book.

Introduction

Why write a book on medical errors and medical malpractice?

In today's society, it is difficult to pick up a newspaper or watch a television show without seeing an ad or a commercial concerning the current malpractice crisis that we have in the United States. Indeed, medical malpractice has become an issue of concern for more than the physicians and plaintiff attorneys. Insurance companies are either ceasing to offer medical malpractice insurance or charging exorbitant amounts in order to cover the enormous amounts awarded by the courts. Politicians are receiving pressure from the medical community to pass reforms limiting 'pain and suffering' damages. Hospital administrators must deal with many physicians forfeiting their privileges and not providing emergency room coverage. Furthermore, hospitals are being forced to revise their by-laws to keep physicians who are now going 'bare' because they cannot afford malpractice insurance. Finally, the most important part of our society – the general public – has been and will continue to be affected, as access to healthcare, and particularly specialists, becomes limited. Therefore it is easy to understand why any literature that addresses this topic would be of paramount importance.

Should we practice 'defensive medicine'?

This is an extremely difficult question to answer. The general conception among the public, and even among some healthcare providers, is that defensive medicine is utilization of 'every test and consultant available' in order to 'not miss something.' The term 'CYA' – 'cover your ass' – has sometimes become synonymous with defensive medicine. In fact, some may even believe that defensive medicine restricts the 'thinking process' and is 'bad medicine.' In this sense, defensive medicine raises the cost burden of healthcare and should not be practiced.

However, defensive medicine also means defending your patient from potential harm to life and limb based on her complaints. This harm can come acutely (acute appendicitis), subacutely (stable angina becoming unstable), or even years from the initial visit (development of breast cancer). For the prudent physician, this means getting a detailed history, performing a thorough exam, formulating a differential diagnosis, ordering the appropriate tests, giving the best treatment, and ensuring that proper instructions and follow-up are given. It does not necessarily mean that more tests and increased healthcare costs are going to occur with every patient. We give many examples in the book where this is not the case. Utilizing telephone consultations with specialists, peer review of charts, and patient callbacks are some methods that are not costly or regarded as 'bad medicine.'

Furthermore, defensive medicine entails that the physician constantly contemplates in her mind what she might be missing or what unexpected outcome could result from each decision that she makes. This is not to say the physician should practice medicine with paranoia of making a mistake; instead, it is a reminder for the physician to stay alert and broad-minded during the decision process. This concept also applies to and should be reflected in the chart documentation. To give an example used by many other authors, the physician should frequently imagine herself in the courtroom with the plaintiff lawyer asking why she did or did not do something or if she had ever considered the 'other' possibilities of the problem. Alternatively, the physician can picture herself in the courtroom staring at her progress note enlarged to a 24 by 36 inch poster and having to explain it.

Once again, we are not advocating that physicians should practice in fear to avoid the courtroom; we are only encouraging our colleagues to be aware of the ramifications of their actions and decisions. This does not necessarily equate to ordering more tests or consultations but it does mandate that examinations and documentations are more thorough and complete in thought. In this manner, defensive medicine not only benefits the physicians legally, but more importantly, it serves the best interests of the patients by guiding physicians to honor one of their Hippocratic oaths – 'do no harm.'

Goals of this book

We believe that there has never been a better time for a book like this to be published. It is written with the intention of providing physicians with a guide for performing and documenting medicine that will decrease the chances of a poor outcome for the patient and for the physician in the courtroom. Physicians should take a proactive approach clinically to avoid contributing to the medical malpractice dilemma. Although there will always be, and always should be, medical malpractice cases in the United States, we believe that physicians will be able to decrease the nontrivial and especially the trivial cases. It is our goal to reach primary care providers, urgent care providers, and emergency providers because their clinical scenarios are where we have based our experiences. However, we believe other groups that may derive benefit and foresight from this book are the senior medical students and young medical residents. They are the ones that we can inform and influence early in their careers about the realities of current medical practice with the goal of instilling good practice habits.

Our hope is to provide the reader with a mindset to practice thorough and sound medicine and minimize medical liability. Although it is not feasible or recommended to use every concept that we have included in this book on each patient encounter, it is left to the reader's discretion as to what would be best for each particular patient. However, remember that you will usually not have the opportunity to make additions at a later time. We have included methods and techniques that we have learned from years of clinical practice in various different clinical settings (e.g. private office, private emergency department, government emergency department, academic residency centers, and as legal consultant for the State Board of Health). In addition, we have a great interest in medical-legal literature that, as of the printing of this book, is still scarcely authored by physicians. From our enthusiastic reading of medical-legal cases, we have tried to incorporate interesting and educational cases into this book to illustrate our concepts. We must also credit our colleagues through the years with sharing their stories (some of which we have used in this book).

We hope that our readers enjoy reading this book as much as we enjoyed writing it. Although the topic of medical malpractice is not a favorite subject of discussion among physicians, we hope that this book will generate an increase in physician interest and discussions concerning legal medicine. Therefore, we encourage our readers to provide us with feedback on our concepts and send us additional techniques that they may use in their own practice.

Chapter 1 is devoted to the progress note. As physicians, we have read many books and listened to multiple mentors instruct us on the contents of a progress note. Medical notes were traditionally only reviewed by healthcare providers. Their purpose was to document the clinical findings. However, today's medical records are increasingly reviewed by non-medical personnel such as attorneys, managed care company representatives, and state licensing agencies. Therefore we must make adjustments in our traditional style of documentation.

Chapter 2 is a brief summary of Chapter 1. In addition, we discuss some other forms of documentation that may be placed in the patient's chart. These additional forms of documentation include patient messages, pharmacy calls, physician phone calls, leaving against medical advice forms, and refusal of care forms. Finally, we reinforce the importance of thorough documentation in decreasing your medical liability.

Chapter 3 focuses on the subjects that should not be placed in the progress note. We purposely placed this chapter immediately after the chapters on the progress note because we feel that it is equally important. Much of what is discussed of this chapter is not taught in medical schools (to some extent, even in residency training) but is largely learned through clinical practice. We present examples of high-risk documentation that we have acquired from personal experience and literature review.

Chapter 4 continues the discussion of high-risk medical activities. This chapter extends beyond the progress note to cover more of clinical practice and judgment. Specifically, it focuses on things that clinicians should avoid doing in their practices. Most of the topics in this chapter are acquired through personal experience and literature review. Very little of this topic is found in medical reference texts or taught in medical schools.

Chapter 5 presents various types of 'difficult patients' and how they may contribute to increasing the physician's medical liability. We offer our experience in dealing with these types of patients and discuss what has worked well for us. Through our experiences in the emergency department and the private office, we have encountered myriad human personalities that have prepared us in writing this chapter. The wonderful aspect of a chapter like this is that it will never be complete because every patient encounter that a physician has in her career is different from any previous one. We welcome our readers to send us ideas and suggestions for further writings.

Chapters 6 and 7 are clinically oriented chapters that offer tips to decrease liability in your practice. These tips cover a very broad scope including office practice, education, personal life, personality, mannerisms, and relationships. We extracted much of the information in this chapter from numerous medical-legal books that we have read, in an effort to share it with our colleagues.

Chapter 8 is entitled 'Things that may go wrong (but are out of your control).' From the title, one may conclude that the ideas in this chapter are not as important to be aware of. However, we had much fun in writing this chapter and thought it would be interesting to insert it in the book. External factors that we have no or little control of are part of everyone's (not just a physician's) daily life. Although we may not be able to change these factors, we still feel that physicians will benefit by being aware of their presence because of the high amount of legal activity involved with our profession. Again, we welcome our readers sending us ideas and suggestions for additional writings.

Chapters 9 and 10 concern legal issues involving emergency physicians. Many of the topics in this chapter are ubiquitous in the practice of emergency medicine and entail legal implications. Patient dumping, abuse, and patient protection are some of the issues discussed. We also provide many clinical cases and discussions.

The book concludes with a chapter that discusses events that occur after a physician is sued. These events are unpleasant for those who have experienced it and even bothersome to those who have not experienced it. Nevertheless, it is a process that we feel every physician should be aware of and be prepared for. The chapter also contains examples of what to do and what not to do in the litigation process.

As a final note, our second book, *Learning from Medical Errors: clinical problems* is also published by Radcliffe Publishing. This book discusses medical errors and legal problems involved in common complaints that lead to malpractice claims. A case presentation and discussion format is also used.

The progress note

- Chief complaint
- History of Present Illness
- Past medical history
- Social history
- Current medications
- Allergies
- Family history
- Surgical history
- Gynecological history
- Review of systems
- Vital signs
- Physical exam
- Differential diagnosis
- Labs/tests
- Hospital/office course
- Consultations
- Assessment
- Plan (with condition at discharge)

The progress note is to the physician what a canvas is to the painter. It is a medium for the physician to document his particular encounter with a patient. It is a permanent document that is used by the treating physician and other physicians as a basis of reference, by plaintiff attorneys in litigation cases, and by hospital review committees for quality and assurance. The physician must be neat, clearly descriptive, and non-offensive in his presentation. The physician must also show logical deductive and reasoning abilities in his decisions.

Chief complaint

This section belongs solely to the patient. The patient's main problem(s) should be stated in his own words. Refrain from using pre-assigned diagnoses here like 'UTI,' 'Stroke,' 'Hypoglycemia,' etc., because it may be assumed that you are predetermining the patient's problem, particularly if the patient or nurse writes something different as the complaint. For example, if the patient writes as the reason for visit – burning and frequency with urination, and you write as the chief complaint 'UTI,' it may be argued by a plaintiff attorney whether you considered other potential causes such as vaginitis, bladder prolapse, etc. Also, be aware of what the patient's complaints are because they must be addressed during the visit and a therapeutic solution should be derived for each complaint. Quite frequently, we will see progress notes with multiple complaints, and one or two of those are never addressed in the note. Even if you do not have time to address a particular complaint, document your reason for believing that it does not need to be acutely addressed and what disposition you gave the patient for this complaint (e.g. having the patient bring it up at the next visit, having the patient see a consultant, telling the patient you will research it, etc.). The rule of thumb here is to never let the patient leave your office feeling that you did not read his or her reason for coming to see you. It not only exposes you to potential liability but also does not lead to good patient rapport.

History of Present Illness (HPI)

This section consists of contributions from multiple sources (the patient, the doctor's questions, family members, friends, paramedics, etc.). Its purpose is to create a more detailed chronologic story concerning the patient's complaint(s). This section is, in our opinion, the most important component of the progress note for multiple reasons. It is the physician's first opportunity to obtain information that will form his basis for decision making during the rest of the visit. It will dictate the questions to ask in the past medical history, family history, social history, and review of systems. It will also suggest which systems to address during the physical exam. Furthermore, the HPI starts the thought process towards formulating a differential diagnosis.

We are all familiar with asking the different qualities of a symptom during the HPI (e.g. onset, duration, severity, quality, modifying factors, associated symptoms, etc.). However, the HPI is an important component of the progress note because the physician can and should include any data that pertains to the chief complaint in this section. This data can be extremely important in multiple aspects (e.g. previous tests for the same complaint, family history of similar complaints, recent changes in social history that may lead to or affect the complaint, etc.). Asking additional questions like these not only enables a physician to obtain additional insight and better treat the patient, but also demonstrates to all potential reviewers of the chart that the thought process included factors surrounding the complaint.

Case 1.1 Build your evaluation from previous ones

An 84-year-old female came to our emergency department (ED) complaining of constant, dull, chest pain across her lower chest for six weeks. The patient had a history of coronary artery disease and had coronary artery angioplasty 10 years ago. This pain, however, was different because it was worse with deep breaths and did not radiate to her arms or jaw.

We proceeded to ask her more about her history of this present illness. She had been vacationing in Florida from New York City for the winter and had been to four different emergency departments (including ours) for this same complaint. This included a visit to another hospital in our city the previous night where she was upset with the ED physician. That physician

continued

told her that he could not do anything for her chronic pain and discharged her. She also said that chest X-rays and electrocardiograms were the only tests that were done on her previous three ED visits. She felt that the physicians had never asked her about the prior visits and, subsequently, they all ran the same tests. 'They also all gave me pain medicines that do not work.' She further added that she had smoked five packs of cigarettes per day for approximately 40 years.

Upon listening to her story, our immediate impression was that she warranted a step-up in care. We proceeded to perform a full cardiac evaluation and also ordered a chest CT and pulmonary study to evaluate her pain. The cardiac tests were unremarkable as expected. The CT scan, however, showed bilateral cavitary pulmonary masses with widespread metastases to the liver, the mediastinum, and the ribs. There was also prominent adenopathy of the hilum and the axillary area. These findings were consistent with those of bronchogenic carcinoma. We admitted her to the hospital for pain management and an oncologic evaluation. She was grateful that someone had finally listened to her.

To reiterate, any new complaint that is brought up in this section must be addressed. Indeed, this is a common theme of any new problem that arises during the patient encounter. As we will discuss in the 'Plan' section, the task of addressing multiple problems need not be as tedious as you may believe at this time.

In the event the patient is a poor historian, not able to give a history, or may be giving a false history, it is helpful to document an alternate history from someone (e.g. family member, neighbor, accident witness, etc.) who might be able to give you another perspective. Should no one be available, document this and any attempt to reach another source that you might have made. One particular case in point that we frequently encounter in Florida is the patient that speaks another language besides English. Here, the physician should make every attempt to find an interpreter because there are potential liability issues when he just writes, 'the patient speaks no English.' Rules may vary among regions and facilities. However, 'patients with limited English have a legal right, through Title VI legislation, to free interpreter services if the institution receives federal money of any type.'[1] In this scenario, a physician would be held accountable for missing a diagnosis because he did not obtain an adequate history.

The physician should not only utilize the HPI to elicit more associated details of the chief complaint(s), he should also emphasize the pertinent details that are not associated with the chief complaint(s). Including the pertinent negatives in the HPI enables the physician to narrow the list of diagnostic possibilities and displays a deductive reasoning process to anyone who reviews the chart.

The important thing to remember about the HPI is that it will probably be the most useful reference if you get sued. In general, the details of a lawsuit are usually discussed 1–2 years after the events have occurred. For the patient involved, this event is a rather drastic and unusual event for him and he should have no problems remembering the fine details of the visit and his conversations with you. For the physician, however, this visit may not, until now, have particularly stood out from the hundreds to thousands of patient encounters that he has had in the past 1–2 years. Therefore, it is more likely that the physician's recollection of the data will be dependent on his 'story of the illness' (in other words, the HPI). Hence, the importance of thorough documentation here cannot be overstated.

One final word of advice with the HPI is that the clinician should always prefer written proof to the patient's verbal statement. We will provide an example to demonstrate how relying on the patient's history without attempting to confirm it will get one in trouble. The second example we will save until the 'Social history' section.

Case 1.2 Differences in terminology

We saw an elderly female in the emergency room for chest pain. When she was asked if she had ever had a heart catheterization, she replied that she had one last year at another hospital and was told that it was 'okay.' Based on this presumption, our plan was to discharge her if her heart tests returned negative. However, we were suspicious because there are not many elderly women with 'normal' coronaries, so we faxed a request for the catheterization report. Her tests came back negative and we kept the patient an additional hour while waiting for the report. Indeed, the wait was well worth it as the report revealed that she had 90% stenosis of one of her coronaries. This revelation turned our disposition plans a complete 180 degrees and left us wondering what could have happened had she been discharged based on inaccurate information.

Of course, there will be situations where getting previous reports or objective confirmation of a history is not possible or practical (e.g. place of testing is closed, data stored in hospital warehouse, old chart is missing, etc.) In these cases, document any attempt that you made and why it failed. This demonstrates to future chart reviewers that you gave your best effort and were left with the patient's stated history as the source of information.

Past medical history

In this section, the physician obtains information on any medical problems that the patient has that might be related to the chief complaint(s). The first assessment the physician should make is whether the patient has a prior history of the current complaint. While this information should be placed in the HPI, it should also be included here as a reminder. If the patient has had similar problems in the past, it will helpful to note how it was or is treated. Next, the physician should ascertain whether the patient has any medical problems that may be related to the chief complaint. An example would be to ask if there is a history of diabetes in someone who presents with an acute infection. We know of a case where a plaintiff attorney had a client who suffered a non-healing wound on his toe because the patient continued to smoke and worsened his peripheral vascular disease. The plaintiff attorney focused his arguments at the deposition on whether the physician asked the patient if he was a diabetic. Finally, the physician should inquire about medical conditions that may be worsened from the presenting complaint. Anticipating the worsening of diabetes because a patient cannot hold down his or her medicine due to the complaint of nausea and vomiting is an expectation of a good physician.

The importance of the past medical history was evident in a recent case that we had.

Case 1.3 Do not let the past haunt you

An elderly woman presented to the ED with the complaint of right chest pain for 24 hours. It was not associated with shortness of breath, radiation to the jaw or arms, diaphoresis, nausea, or vomiting. The ED physician who saw her ordered an electrocardiogram and cardiac enzymes, which were all negative. He then went off shift and told the oncoming physician that he did not know what the etiology was but that he did not feel that it was cardiac in nature. He also recommended that the patient be discharged if the chest X-ray was unremarkable.

The oncoming physician reviewed the chart and noticed that the only listing in the past medical history section was 'leg fracture.' After looking at the chest X-ray and not being impressed with it, he proceeded to see the patient. She had early Alzheimer's dementia and was a poor historian. The physician lifted the sheets and saw that her right lower leg was in a cast. This made the physician consider pulmonary embolus as a cause of this patient's pain. He felt it was unlikely, though, because her oxygen saturation was 97% on room air, her pain was not pleuritic, and she was not complaining of shortness of breath. However, there were enough doubts in his mind that he ordered a spiral CT scan of the chest and pulmonary vessels. The scan showed large bilateral pulmonary emboli with right ventricular strain as evidenced by deviation of the interventricular septum. The legs were also scanned with the CT and deep venous thromboses were seen in both legs.

Social history

Many physicians commonly overlook this section of the progress note. Although we were taught the value of this section in medical school and how it would help us understand the patient's environment, we clinically often suppress this section to one or two casual and routine questions. Effective use of social history can provide information on the patient's occupation, habits, cultural beliefs, living environment, living will status, etc. The questions to ask depend on the patient's presenting complaint.

For a patient who presents with a worker's compensation injury, the patient's occupation and tasks required while on duty should be included. In someone with chest pain, tobacco use or cocaine use becomes important. The bleeding patient needs to be asked if he is a Jehovah's Witness. The head injury patient should not be sent home if he lives alone or cannot be under the supervision of a responsible adult. Finally, the critically ill patient's resuscitation wishes must be known for proper care.

Here is an example of using discretion with the information that patients may give you. We have seen at least a handful of healthy young males (less than 30 years of age) who presented to us with new-onset seizures, but who adamantly denied that they used any illicit drugs. We performed full evaluations and found that every test is negative with the exception of positive urine drug screens (usually for cocaine). Whether or not the drug is the responsible culprit is debatable, but suspicion of common etiologies (especially in this patient population) should always be maintained despite the patient's denial.

The final comment concerning social history is that the patient's living conditions are extremely important in certain complaints. Seizure patients who drive an automobile or operate machinery need to be instructed not to do so. Patients without transportation or who live far away should have a lower threshold for admission because of their increased difficulty in returning for medical evaluation. Elderly patients and pediatric patients should have responsible caregivers who can follow discharge instructions (e.g. be hesitant about discharging a febrile pediatric patient of unknown etiology to a teenage, first-time mother). Remember that your responsibility for the patient's medical illness does not end once they leave your office or emergency department and that the public's (lawyers', judge's, jury's) expectations are that you anticipate obstacles that may prevent the patient either from returning if the conditions worsen, or from following the necessary instructions for clinical improvement.

Current medications

Ideally, this section should include all of the patient's prescription and non-prescription medications. Medication dosages should also be noted. Alternative therapeutic modalities such as oxygen, continuous positive airway pressure (CPAP), herbal medicines, and physical therapy should also be included. We all know from clinical experience that medicines and dosages are difficult to memorize. Therefore, ideal conditions are often not met. In these situations, the physician must use his ingenuity. In the office, it is always helpful to keep an updated list of medications and dosages on the front cover of the chart. If you use this practice, you should still include this section in each progress note with a comment of where to find the current medications. This technique reminds you to address this section as patients can be taking new over-the-counter medicines or prescription medicines from another physician without your awareness. This technique is also helpful should someone else review your progress note without access to the rest of the chart. They would then know where to obtain the list.

In the emergency department, old charts, admission notes, or discharge summaries can be retrieved. Familiarity with the patient's medications has an additional benefit in the emergency department. With the convenience of having a laboratory and being able to do blood work, we are able to check levels of common medications like digoxin, Dilantin, phenobarbital, Tylenol, and aspirin. Because these levels are frequently helpful in ED evaluations, it is prudent to ask the patient if he is specifically taking any of these medications.

Other sources you could utilize to obtain the medications that your patients are taking include pharmacies, family members, and nursing homes. Good charting entails consistent updating of medication lists and documentation of attempts at getting them.

Allergies

In the event of an adverse drug reaction, the medical and legal implications in omitting this section from the progress note are enormous. There will be no legal defense for the physician who prescribes a known allergic medicine to a patient without first asking the patient. If you feel that there are few alternative medicines for the patient, then ask and document what their exact reaction is. The reaction may have been a side effect or intolerance and not a true allergy. If the patient is allergic to a particular medicine (e.g. Toradol) and you would like to give an anti-inflammatory for gout, ask if they have taken another medicine from that family (e.g. ibuprofen). If they have safely taken another medicine from the same family of drugs, then you should document this in the chart and you will probably be safe in administering it.

Family history

This section must be individualized for each patient and/or each complaint. Inquire about coronary artery disease in patients with chest pain, asthma in patients with wheezing, peptic ulcer disease in patients with gastrointestinal bleeding, and aneurysms in patients with headaches, etc. Certain patient groups that may be particularly susceptible to certain diseases should also receive specific questioning. Does the African-American patient have sickle cell disease in the family? Does the tall, thin patient with chest pain have Marfan's syndrome in the family? These are all pertinent questions to include in specific groups of patients.

In the emergency setting, two common areas of medical liability are the chest pain patient and the headache patient. Chest pain patients with family history have an additional risk factor for coronary artery disease and should be taken more seriously than those with negative family history. We have seen a couple handfuls of patients that were under 35 years of age with acute myocardial infarctions and no cardiac risk factors with the exception of family history. Unfortunately, we have also seen a few of these discharged home with acute myocardial infarction because their family history was not taken seriously.

> ### Case 1.4 Do not minimize family ties
>
> We recently saw a patient in the emergency department who returned after she was treated four days prior in the ED for a migraine. She was 36 years old and did not have a history of headaches but did have a family history of brain aneurysms. Her CT scan showed a subacute subarachnoid hemorrhage.

For the primary care physician, a family history of cancer has frequently played a role in medical malpractice cases.

Case 1.5 Dig up family secrets

Our friend was sued by a 40-year-old gentleman who was diagnosed with late-stage colon cancer from a colonoscopy performed for rectal bleeding. The patient claimed that the physician should have inquired about his family history because his father had colon cancer and, thus performed colon cancer screening earlier. The patient stated that these interventions would have drastically improved his prognosis. Our friend, however, noted that the patient did not admit on his previous visits that there were any medical problems in his family. The specific questioning for cancer in the family was not documented. The case is still pending. A similar sequence of events is also commonly seen with breast cancer.

Some family physicians have developed preprinted sheets with a checklist of diseases for the patient to check off. We find that this will save time and decrease liability. We like to add a write-in section for diseases that are not included on the checklist. The important concept to remember is to not underestimate the significance of a family history.

Surgical history

This is another section that is often overlooked and, for most complaints is probably unnecessary. Including the surgical history is extremely valuable to the diagnostic evaluation and therapeutic intervention for certain complaints. The classic example is the patient with abdominal pain. In *Emergency Medicine: concepts and clinical practice* we find: 'prior surgeries are important for many reasons. For example, almost 70% of patients with small bowel obstruction have had previous abdominal surgery.'[2] Hence, knowledge of what abdominal surgeries a patient has had will give you an idea of his risk for bowel obstruction, adhesions, or possible recurrent problems (e.g. perforated peptic ulcer, diverticulitis), and it will also narrow the differential diagnosis by eliminating organs that have been removed.

Noting previous surgical scars will aid greatly in the medical history of a patient that may not be able to give you a history. A midline chest scar could suggest coronary artery disease and a previous coronary artery bypass graft. A midline abdominal scar might suggest peripheral vascular disease and an abdominal aortic aneurysm repair. Finally, a left upper quadrant scar may mean that the spleen was removed and the patient is more susceptible to certain infections such as those with encapsulated organisms.

Finally, inquiring about recent surgery can be helpful in certain groups of patients. Some examples would include the patient with suspected deep venous thrombosis from non-ambulation, the patient with fevers and shortness of breath from atelectasis, and the patient with constipation from narcotics. Knowledge of what surgery the patient has had will also give you a hint to look for its complications. A good example would be the patient with a gastrointestinal hemorrhage from an aortic-intestinal fistula as a complication of abdominal aortic aneurysm repair.

Gynecologic history

This section is usually divided into several subsections and is appropriate to include in any female with an abdominal or gynecologic (e.g. breast, pelvic) complaint. It should consist of the pregnancy history (i.e. gravity, parity, blood type, and any pregnancy complications), the gynecologic history (i.e. last menstrual period, history of fibroids, history of ovarian cysts, last mammogram, and history of breast disease), and the sexual history (i.e. previous STDs, forms of contraception used, and history of pelvic inflammatory disease). Gynecologic surgeries could also be included here or in the surgical section.

The information obtained in this section is essential to the evaluation of lower abdominal pain in females due to the proximity of the gynecologic organs to the gastrointestinal organs. A classic example would be a female presenting with a small bowel obstruction caused by adhesions from previous gynecologic surgeries. Note that upper abdominal pain may also sometimes be of gynecologic origin such as in the case of Fitz-Hugh–Curtis syndrome. We have experienced that the majority of females do not consider gynecologic surgeries as abdominal surgeries; therefore, if you did not take a gynecologic history in someone who had a vaginal hysterectomy, you may not be on the alert for a bowel obstruction in your evaluation.

Another portion of the gynecologic history often omitted is the last menstrual period. We have found that this data has significant contributions to the patient with right lower quadrant pain. While the clinical findings of acute appendicitis may be similar to pelvic inflammatory disease, if the appendix is normal on CT scan and the patient is currently on her period, the diagnosis of pelvic inflammatory disease becomes much more likely.

Review of systems

This section gives the physician an opportunity to elicit the pertinent positives and negatives of different organ systems as it pertains to the chief complaint(s). We have found it best to go through this section systematically (i.e. head to toe), so that you will be less likely to skip over an organ system. Think of it as an extension of the HPI where you are able to obtain more details of the presenting complaint and narrow your working diagnosis.

Along with the typical organ systems, we like to include a 'constitutional' system where we can ask for fevers, weight loss, fatigue, etc. We feel that the presence of fever is probably the most important review of system element to ascertain because of its relevance to almost every complaint. Furthermore, its presence can and should alert the physician to a more serious etiology. For example, the complaint of headache usually does not demand an extensive work-up; however, in the presence of fever, meningitis or encephalitis becomes higher on the differential.

The second example where fever can change the list of differential diagnoses comes in back pain. Again, the complaint of back pain usually does not warrant an extensive evaluation. However, when back pain is accompanied by fevers, other serious etiologies such as epidural abscess or osteomyelitis must be considered. In the low back pain chapter in our companion book, *Learning from Medical Errors: clinical problems*, we present a case of an epidural abscess (**Case 7.2**) and a case of diskitis (**Case 7.3**).

It is prudent to reiterate that any new findings derived from this section need to be addressed in the evaluation. If the findings appear to be unrelated to the chief complaint and have little acute significance, then you should simply acknowledge the findings and assure a referral for future evaluation. However, not addressing a positive finding can have grave consequences in the future.

Case 1.6 Remember what the patient said

One of our colleagues endured this unfortunate scenario a few years ago. He was performing a routine physical in which the patient stated that he had seen some spots of blood in his stool. The patient had a history of hemorrhoids so he was treated for such. Two years later, he was diagnosed with colon cancer and filed a lawsuit against the physician for not initiating an earlier work-up for rectal bleeding.

Vital signs

Always request that vital signs are obtained at every visit (except maybe the suture removal, the PPD check, etc.). Furthermore, we prefer to have the vital signs completed before we see the patient so that we can develop a quick mental picture in our mind and address any abnormal vital sign with the patient. The standard four vital signs include: pulse, blood pressure, respiratory rate, and temperature.[3] We like the addition of the 'fifth vital sign', pulse oximetry, if you have the equipment. Vital signs are important in that they are an inexpensive, quick, objective method of evaluating the patient's illness. The adage 'vital signs don't lie' is a double-edged sword. While it is frequently helpful in the patient who cannot give a history or gives a false history, it also asserts loudly to everyone who reviews the chart that 'if I am abnormal I need to be addressed and explained.'

Think twice about discharging someone if you cannot explain the stability of an abnormal vital sign or document its improvement after treatment. Make a habit of recording multiple sets of vital signs when the initial set is abnormal or the patient's condition is likely to change during the visit. This demonstrates acknowledgment of the abnormal vital sign and your subsequent intervention and monitoring. At the extreme, it is recommended to record vital signs every three minutes in the early stages of a trauma.[4] Depending on where you practice medicine, be cognizant of the 'standard of care' among physicians in your area concerning abnormal vital signs. After all, your local colleagues are likely to be the expert witnesses for plaintiff attorneys. For example, in our emergency department, we do not discharge infants and toddlers until their temperature is below 103°F because of the risk for febrile seizures.

We request that pulse oximetry, at the minimum, be performed in any patient presenting with chest symptoms, abdominal symptoms (pneumonia presenting as abdominal pain), or upper airway symptoms. Our experience is that this vital sign (along with blood pressure) is a tough one to gauge clinically. Although you can usually feel if a patient is febrile, get a rough estimate of the respiratory rate and heart rate by touching and looking at the patient, we are often fooled by the pulse oximetry. We have particularly found some pneumonias masquerading as abdominal pain by recognizing a patient's low oxygen saturation.

Also keep in mind that there are variations of vital signs that may be useful in certain situations, to help you clinically make a diagnosis and also to legally suggest against a particular diagnosis. Common examples would be orthostatic blood pressure in the patient with dizziness or taking blood pressures in both arms in the patient with chest pain and suspected aortic dissection.

Case 1.7 Simple clue goes a long way

We had an interesting case where the recording of blood pressure in both arms led to an unsuspected diagnosis. A 64-year-old man came to our ED with upper back pain. The pain was nontraumatic and had been present for four months. He was seen by his primary physician and another ED during this time and had numerous tests. These included X-rays of the thoracic spine and a gallbladder ultrasound. Both of the tests were unremarkable. The pain was occasionally associated with numbness in his right arm. He had a history of hypertension and heavy tobacco use.

The blood pressure in his left arm was 160/94 mm Hg and his physical exam was unremarkable. Our initial impression was that he probably had a 'bulging disk' in his neck or upper back. However, we were concerned about an aortic dissection with the patient's past medical history and tobacco use. Hence, we asked the nurse to obtain a blood pressure in the patient's right arm. This was 105/70 mm Hg. A similar discrepancy occurred when the blood pressures were repeated. This finding heightened our suspicion and we ordered a Computed Tomography (CT) scan of the patient's chest.

The CT scan did not reveal an aortic dissection. Instead, it gave us a surprising etiology for the patient's symptoms and blood pressure discrepancy. He had a thrombosed clot in his right subclavian artery. There were also clots in his superior mesenteric artery and his inferior mesenteric artery. The patient was started on anticoagulants and admitted to the vascular surgery service.

The next case is an unfortunately sad one that might have been prevented had a complete set of vitals been recorded. We worked with an emergency nurse who was notorious for taking shortcuts when he was assigned to perform triage duties. Despite working with him for four years and repeated reminders to him to obtain all vitals in every patient, he never seemed to make it standard practice. We would persistently hear resistant questioning from this nurse. Why do we need pulse oximetry in abdominal pain? Why do we need blood pressure in someone with a sore throat? However, we discovered that it was not only the subtle cases that he would question but he would omit vital signs in obvious cases, too. For example, patients with shortness of breath and cough would not have a temperature taken or patients with light-headedness would not have a blood pressure recorded.

Case 1.8 A fatal omission

This nurse triaged an 80-year-old man one day who came in with right hip pain after falling on it. The patient had a history of chronic obstructive pulmonary disease and had one lung removed. The nurse took all of his vitals but did not feel that a pulse oximetry was needed for a probable hip fracture. The emergency physician saw the chart and noticed that all the vitals were unremarkable (with the exception of an omitted pulse oximetry) and ordered a hip X-ray.

After the X-ray confirmed a fracture of the femoral neck, the orthopedist was called to admit the patient. Orders were given to move the patient to the operating suite. As the patient was ready to be moved from the ED, the nurse recorded one final set of vitals. When the patient was placed on the monitor a pulse oximetry of 40% appeared on the screen. The nurse saw this but did not believe the reading because 'the patient was talking to me.' There was a nursing change of shift before the patient was transported. The nurse told the oncoming nurse about the pulse oximetry but that 'it was not real.' He also did not bring it to the ED physician's attention.

As the anesthesiologist saw the patient, he noted the patient's pulse oximetry. He immediately called the orthopedist who wanted the patient to be moved to a critical care area and receive an immediate medical consult. Unfortunately, the only critical care bed available in the hospital was the emergency department. Therefore, the patient was transported back to the ED three hours later.

In the ED, the internist and pulmonologist saw the patient immediately and placed the patient on prophylactic Lovenox. One hour later, the patient had a run of supraventricular tachycardia that was treated with adenosine. Another hour later, the patient suddenly lost consciousness and went into cardiopulmonary arrest. He was unable to be resuscitated. The suspected cause of death was a fat embolus from the hip fracture. We will never know if the fatal events could have been prevented had the first emergency physician been clued in to the patient's respiratory status.

Physical exam

Before you examine the patient, insist that your nurses have the patient undress, at the minimum, the body part involved. Exposure to the natural human body is one of the fundamentals taught to us in physical diagnosis class. Unfortunately, due to time constraints, respect for patient's privacy, or a nurse's or a physician's indolent behavior, we sometimes perform exams through the patient's clothes. There are obvious limitations to this manner of physical examination. Visual inspections for rashes, wounds, bruises, and scars are prohibited. Both the auscultation and the percussion of organs are limited by the thickness of the patient's clothes. Finally, palpation for pulses will be difficult through clothing.

There are other disadvantages to examining a dressed patient. External clothing markers or jewelry may show up on X-rays and be misinterpreted as foreign bodies. Clothing may discourage the physician from examining nearby body areas (e.g. pelvic and genital area in the patient with lower abdominal pain), which could be a source of referred pain. In addition, the patient may feel that he or she is getting an incomplete and hurried exam. We have heard a lot of patients complain that their doctor listened to their lungs through their clothing and did not ask them to undress. Indeed, some patients will get the perception that they spent more time with their physician just by the fact that they had to get into a gown. While some patients may feel uneasy to undress for you, we have found that very few will object when you explain to them that it is the best way for you to examine them.

We have three cases in the ED where we were extremely embarrassed that we did not undress our patients and one case in the office where we were pleased that we did. The first involved an inmate who presented with abdominal pain.

Case 1.9 Hands-on experience

The patient had on ankle cuffs which made it difficult for him to take off his pants so a genital exam was deferred. The abdominal exam and X-ray were consistent with a small bowel obstruction and the patient stated that he did not have a history of hernias. When the surgeon came, he had the patient remove his pants and the patient had a huge incarcerated inguinal hernia. Simply undressing the patient would have saved us much embarrassment. Also, this incident supports the above statement that clothing will discourage you from examining a patient adequately.

Case 1.10 I forgot to look

The second embarrassment came with a man who presented for hemoptysis. He stated that he had a history of aneurysm repair and told us that it was a chest aneurysm. We examined him through a gown and did not pay attention to where his surgical scar was. We sent him for a chest CT to check for an aortic-tracheal fistula. No fistula was seen and the CT was helpful in also ruling out pulmonary embolus or masses. However, when the radiologist commented that there was no evidence of surgery in the chest, we reluctantly had the patient remove his robe to see a large scar in his abdomen and none in his chest.

Case 1.11 A picture is worth a thousand words

Now for the case where we were rewarded for removing the patient's gown. We had seen an elderly lady with a history of coronary artery disease in the office with 'burning pain' in her left chest that radiated around to the back for four days. With her heart history, our impression was to send the patient to the ED for further evaluation. However, when she removed her gown, she had vesicles in a linear distribution exactly where she was describing

continued

the pain. With this finding, an EKG that did not show any change, and the patient stating that this pain did not feel like her prior heart pain and was not associated with diaphoresis, nausea, or vomiting, we felt comfortable in treating her shingles and discharging her with close follow-up.

Case 1.12 Falling for the same mistake twice

As if missing a diagnosis once was not enough, we made the same mistake twice. A 70-year-old lady presented to our ED with pain in the right groin and right buttock. The pain had been present for four days and was not associated with any trauma, fevers, nausea, vomiting, diarrhea, or urinary symptoms. She also said that she was having some numbness in her right buttock. She had been to our ED four days ago and had blood work and a CT urogram (without contrast) that were normal. The pain medicine that was prescribed was not controlling her pain.

On physical examination, she was afebrile and was dressed in a hospital gown with her underwear on. The right groin where she was having pain had mild tenderness but no guarding or rebound and no masses. Her pelvic and rectal examinations (performed with her groin covered with a sheet) were unremarkable. We pulled her previous chart and discovered that she had blood work, urinalysis, and a CT urogram, which were all negative.

We repeated her blood work and it was, once again, negative. An abdominal X-ray showed small bowel distention. A CT scan with contrast of the abdomen was performed to rule out small bowel obstruction. Before the results were available, we called the patient's physician to admit her for refractory pain. He examined her with her underwear and gown off and saw a small vesicle and the diagnosis of herpetic zoster was immediately apparent. It is unnecessary to say that it was extremely embarrassing for two ED physicians to miss a simple diagnosis and order two expensive CT scans. Her second CT scan was normal. Please do not let this happen to you.

While we are on the subject of undressing and examining patients, a discussion concerning the medical chaperone is due. A chaperone of the same sex as the patient should always be used for examination of pelvic, genital, and breast areas. This rule has traditionally applied when the physician is the opposite sex to the patient. However, rules when the physician is the same sex as the patient are controversial. The chaperone should be a medically trained employee of the facility and not just a friend who came to see you. Ideally, you should write the initials of the chaperone or ask the chaperone to document the encounter on the chart in the event that his or her presence is questioned at a later date. The belief that as long as you are professional, your patient will not complain is naïve and untrue, as most of us will attest. There are patients who are always searching for reasons to complain, get attention, or even carry out vendettas against physicians.

Case 1.13 An unpleasant but necessary job

We had an experience in the emergency room that demonstrates this. A man with a long history of alcohol abuse and pancreatitis presented to us with abdominal pain and was intoxicated. After we performed the rectal exam, he asked to see the hospital chaplain because he 'felt violated.' In addition, cultural differences may also contribute to beliefs of unprofessional conduct when none actually exists. Also, since we are professionals and public figures, our conduct is constantly under scrutiny by numerous organizations (*see* Chapter 5).

Remember that the sensitivity to examinations of the 'private parts' is extremely varied among people. Some will completely disrobe and cooperate without questions while it is 'like pulling teeth' with others to even touch their bodies. This behavior is certainly understandable when trust has not developed in the relationship. The perception of some patients may also be affected by the media's portrayal of some physicians who have been inappropriate. We recently saw an episode of the TV drama 'ER' where one of the physicians performed an unnecessary breast exam. His colleague later asked him if he had 'tubed' a patient. The term 'tube' is an acronym for 'totally unnecessary breast exam.' In both of our many years of being in medicine, neither one of us has ever heard of the term. We wonder if the producers of the show invented this term in order to generate ratings at the expense of creating paranoia among female patients.

An important component of the physical exam to always include is the 'General' or 'Constitutional' section. The brief, albeit important, comments in this section serve to paint a visual picture of the patient's presentation for all reviewers of the chart. Take, for example, the description of a patient's pain as 'colicky.' This example would portray a patient with moderate, intermittent pain, such as that from cholelithiasis or ureterolithiasis. Use clear, descriptive terms like well-appearing, toxic, no acute distress, playful, agitated, etc. Since this section contains the inaugural remarks of the physical exam, it makes an immediate impact on the patient's condition to the reviewer. The rest of the exam could be entirely normal but a patient described as 'toxic' will still draw concern for a serious medical illness. In contrast, we would be less alarmed at physical findings if the patient appeared 'in no acute distress.' From our experience with thousands of consultant phone conversations through the years, the most reliable question to ask when deciding whether to admit a patient is: 'How does the patient look, do they look sick?'

Noting the general appearance of the patient is especially important in the evaluation of the pediatric patient. In this population, the history and sometimes the physical can be limited, atypical, or misleading. Therefore, an experienced physician's first impression of whether the patient looks ill or not will usually lead to the correct therapeutic decisions. Likewise, the elderly or demented patient encounter can have similar limitations where documentation of the general appearance is essential to the evaluation.

Many physicians dislike performing pelvic and rectal examinations. Most patients, likewise, do not look forward to having these exams. We have heard hundreds of excuses from both parties to avoid these exams. Physicians will cite that the exams take too much time, it is too hard to get a chaperone, the exam adds little to their clinical decisions, or they 'do not know what [they] are feeling.' In addition, we see more physicians pass the burden of these particular exams to their colleagues more commonly than any other part of the medical evaluation. From the patient's perspective, common excuses are that they had the exams done recently, 'my doctor never does these exams,' or 'those exams are not needed.'

Case 1.14 What did this patient expect?

We saw a 21-year-old male in the ED for 'extreme rectal bleeding.' He believed that he had a history of hemorrhoids. We did a rectal exam and did not find any hemorrhoids. He later wrote a letter of complaint to hospital administration stating that a rectal examination was unnecessary. It was his opinion that we should have trusted him that the source of bleeding was the hemorrhoids. We responded to this complaint with copies from numerous medical references citing the standard of care in the evaluation of rectal bleeding.

We have bad news for all of the physicians and patients in the above paragraph. The goal of the medical visit is for the physician to use his medical skills and for the patient to trust this skill in order to find out the etiology of the patient's problem. This goal sometimes includes unpleasant exams and certainly excludes shortcuts for the sake of convenience. These exams are quick and can be performed without the aid of a speculum or anoscope the majority of the time. For most of us, the purposes of these exams are twofold. Medically, we are examining for tenderness, masses, or bleeding. Legally, we want to show that we are thorough clinicians who leave no stone unturned. Obtaining a chaperone is not a problem in our practice. When a skilled medical person (e.g. nurse, medical assistant) is not available, we simply prepare all the equipment ourselves (e.g. KY jelly, hemoccult card, hemoccult solution, vaginal cultures, etc.) and ask an employee of the hospital or clinic (e.g. secretary, housekeeping, billing person, etc.) to serve as a chaperone as long as the patient does not object.

   We believe that physicians should not proclaim that these exams add little to their clinical decision making. Although this statement is probably true and many authors have written that they rarely add to or alter the treatment regimen, we find it unacceptable in the rare instances when the diagnosis is missed because the exam was not performed. How can you justify to yourself and to a jury that you missed a diagnosis because you did not perform an exam that takes no longer than two minutes and does not cost the patient an extra penny? Furthermore, while it is also true that most physicians seldom encounter enough pelvic or rectal pathology to become proficient at these examinations, how is a physician ever to become proficient if he or she does not practice? In addition, some pathology is crystal clear and just waiting for you to be discovered through the exams.

Case 1.15 Not searching for the obvious

We once worked with an emergency physician who never performed pelvic examinations of women with abdominal pain. Subsequently, he had several cases of females presenting with abdominal pain where he missed the diagnosis. Ironically, in all of these cases, he had diagnosed these women with kidney stones. This is surprising because their symptoms were not those that one would classically expect from a kidney stone. One woman had diffuse abdominal pain and no flank pain, another had epigastric pain with diarrhea, while the third had pelvic pain and vaginal discharge. It was not surprising that all three of these women had negative CT scans of the ureters and kidneys. When the first two charts were reviewed, it was discovered that these women were both on their periods during the medical encounter and that their urine was not collected by catheterization.

The third woman came in with diffuse abdominal pain but no flank pain and no hematuria. The physician ordered blood work, which was unremarkable, and a urinalysis, which showed gross blood. He signed the patient off to us as 'a probable kidney stone.' He had ordered a CT of the ureters and kidney to look for the stone and we were to follow this test. We went to see the patient and obtained a further history. She stated that she was having vaginal spotting although she had just finished her last menstrual period two weeks ago. Because she was African-American and had abnormal vaginal bleeding, we asked about a history of uterine fibroids. To this question, she admitted that she was told of this in the past. We proceeded to perform a pelvic examination in which we found an enlarged uterus and vaginal blood on our glove. We wanted to cancel the CT scan at that point but it was too late. To no one's surprise the scan was negative for kidney or ureteral stones. A pelvic ultrasound, however, confirmed our suspicion of uterine fibroids.

This case highlights two important points. The first is the missed diagnosis due to the omission of a key element in the physician examination of abdominal pain in females. This led to an expensive and useless test that also exposed the patient to unnecessary radiation. We find it shocking how some physicians will order 10 CT scans for abdominal pain before they do a single pelvic or rectal exam for abdominal pain. The second learning point is that it did not require the world's greatest gynecologist to perform this exam in order to find useful information. A first year medical student could have looked on his glove and known why this patient had 'blood in her urine.' The final message about pelvic and rectal examinations is that there is no justification in the courtroom for not doing them (unless you do not have fingers).

We sometimes feel that medical students should be taught the serial physical exam(s) and not just the physical exam in the medical evaluation. Our point in making this statement is that the medical evaluation and the potential legal defense of a medical evaluation are often assisted by multiple exams of the patient during the same encounter. Additional information may be obtained when patients are examined in different positions (e.g. checking for benign positional vertigo, subclavian steal, etc.), repeated examinations are used (e.g. checking for evolving surgical abdomen), and after therapeutic interventions (e.g. checking orthostatics after intravenous fluids, asking about chest pain after nitroglycerin, etc.). A patient that has an initial physical finding that may warrant hospital admission should have a repeat exam of that finding and documentation that the finding is improved (or at least stable and unlikely to deteriorate upon leaving) before discharge is considered. Any patient with a worsening physical exam should not be discharged. Lastly, multiple exams by different providers should all be documented.

The final comment on the physical examination is to make sure that you examine (physically touch) every patient. We have seen physicians rely on examinations by other physicians. We have seen other physicians perform evaluations of patients from another room without ever touching the patient. This nonchalant attitude will sometimes lead to misdiagnosis as the following examples show.

Case 1.16 Medicine is a contact science

Edwards, in *The M & M Files*, presents a case of a six-year-old girl that fell on her wrist and was brought to the ED.[5] The triage nurse was opinionated from prior experiences with the patient's parents. Therefore, she wrote on the chart, 'no obvious injuries, complains of some wrist pain.' The physician was having a busy day covering for a provider who called in sick. When he went to see the patient, he talked to the patient from the doorway and said that nothing was wrong.

The child was brought to her pediatrician the following day where an X-ray was ordered. This revealed a buckle fracture of the distal radius. The pediatrician filed a complaint to the vice president of medical affairs at the hospital. The ED physician responded to the complaint by saying that he was extremely busy on that day and had to rely on the nurse's evaluation. He was subsequently dismissed from the hospital several months later. This consequence was a price the physician had to pay for the few seconds saved by not laying his hands on the patient.

Differential diagnosis

This section is usually placed after the history and physical and is where the physician lists his possible diagnoses for the presenting complaint. It is the foundation on which tests are ordered and therapeutic decisions are made. It may or may not include the final diagnosis (assessment) because the evaluation is incomplete at this point. It should, however, always include common emergent conditions for each particular complaint (e.g. myocardial infarction for chest pain, pulmonary embolus for shortness of breath, small bowel obstruction for refractory vomiting, abdominal aortic aneurysm for flank pain, etc.). The reason for this is that there is usually no or minimal harm as a consequence of missing a benign diagnosis. Remember, the plaintiff attorney must show three things in a malpractice case. He must show that the physician had a relationship with the patient or a duty to treat. He must demonstrate that the physician breached this duty and did not follow the standard of care. Finally, he must show that the physician's inappropriate treatment of the patient resulted in harm to the patient.[6] Therefore, the judge and jury will not look favorably on the physician if a missed diagnosis was not listed in the differential diagnosis.

Whenever a malpractice suit is brought against a physician for a missed diagnosis, the physician's defense case can be strengthened by a thorough differential diagnosis. By including the true diagnosis in your differential diagnosis, you will impress the judge and jury with your consideration of its presence. The caveat to this is that you must either perform the specific test(s) that is (are) needed to evaluate each differential diagnosis or state why you feel that the particular differential diagnosis is unlikely (e.g. doubt pulmonary embolus because no hypoxia, no increased alveolar-arterial gradient, no apparent risk factors, normal d-dimer, etc.). Lee J Johnson, a healthcare attorney in New York, agrees with this philosophy. She recommends that 'even if you just considered a test, note it' in an article from *Medical Economics*.[7]

We believe that this section is particularly important in the progress note because it requires the physician to recall everything that he has learned in his medical career and combine that with the new information that he has just obtained from his patient and formulate diagnostic possibilities from this amalgamation of information. We can all reminisce to our medical school days when our mentor's favorite question was 'what do you think this patient has?' At the time, as medical students, this was our time to 'shine' and show off our knowledge. Now, as practicing physicians, the differential diagnosis section gives us a chance to impress the plaintiff lawyers, the judge, and the jury our vast medical knowledge and our extensive clinical experience. With this belief, we would like to see more physicians include this section in their progress notes. Similarly, we are proponents of greater emphasis on this section in teaching medical students on how to write a progress note.

Labs/tests

Physicians should review all labs or tests that are performed in the office or emergency department. When the results are normal or unremarkable, a simple comment that they were 'reviewed' is sufficient. This lets all reviewers know that the clinician was aware of the results. It also serves as a reminder for the physician to follow up on tests that were ordered. We believe that most physicians have ordered tests for which they have lost track. This is particularly true in an emergency setting where one has 15 patients at a time with an average of three to four labs or tests on each patient.

The results of abnormal tests should also be recorded in the chart. It is especially important to display to future and potential chart reviewers that you were fully aware of the abnormal result and that your medical decisions on that patient reflected an understanding of these results. As a general rule, abnormal test results should be reflected in the final diagnoses. Even if the abnormal results have no relation to the patient's presenting complaint, they should be listed as diagnoses in order to be addressed at a future time.

Hospital/office course

This section is not traditionally taught in medical schools or in medical texts. However, we feel that it is extremely important to include it because it serves to testify that the patient/physician encounter is frequently a dynamic interaction that consists of more than a conversation and examination between the physician and the patient. Some patients may require immediate therapeutic or pharmacologic treatments in the office to alter the condition or conditions with which they present. This is particularly true in the emergency department setting, where the majority of patients will receive some form of intervention (e.g. medications, reduction of dislocations, therapeutic or diagnostic procedures such as chest thoracostomy, etc.)

Interventions in the office or emergency department should be documented for several reasons. There should be a permanent record of any intervention in order to assess for improvement or worsening of the presenting condition. If the condition is unchanged or deteriorates with the intervention, accurate documentation may prevent the physician or future providers from using the same intervention. Likewise, if an intervention is successful, future providers may benefit from this knowledge. In the event of an iatrogenic adverse outcome, documentation may indict the provider but, rest assured, the provider will be in a more ominous predicament if there is no such documentation. Chart reviewers may believe that the omission was intentional. Even if you just give the patient a sample of a medication, do not forget to note this, because one pill is all that is need for most reactions to occur.

Interventions can consist of something simple like repeating a blood pressure or a temperature. Documentation of improving vital signs gives an objective sense that the patient's condition is improving. This improvement will be hard for a lawyer to dispute. In contrast, if vital signs improve but were not recorded, the physician will have a heavier burden in court showing that the patient was improved before discharge.

The multi-trauma patient presents an emergency scenario where documentation can become complicated. Here, it is not unusual to have multiple medications administered or multiple procedures performed at the same time. This frenzy of activity makes it easy to forget to document a certain procedure or to document a certain procedure inaccurately. To make matters more difficult, accurate timing of when interventions are performed is mandated in the trauma patient. Therefore, it is helpful to have assistants help you with recording the activities in a trauma.

Repeat physical exams may also be included in this section. In addition, sometimes the patient may develop a totally new problem while waiting for the treatment of the initial problem.

Case 1.17 (also Case 6.12) One thing led to another

We took care of a patient who presented with right lateral rib pain after falling off a motorcycle. He was found to have two right lateral rib fractures. When he started to vomit after being in the emergency

continued

department for two hours, an EKG showed an acute myocardial infarction and 100% occlusion of his left anterior descending artery. The stress and pain from his injury probably provoked his coronary artery disease.

In these situations, it may be confusing to understand the patient's treatment by just reading the initial history and physical if a hospital/office course section is not included.

Consultations

This section should include the names of all consultants that the patient's case was discussed with during the visit along with the time of the consultation. Consultants include physicians, home health nurses, dieticians, pharmacists, and other healthcare professionals. In addition, consultants may also consist of family members, employers, witnesses, etc. The name of the consultant and an extremely brief synopsis of the conversation should be recorded on the chart.

Case 1.18 Getting everyone on the same page

Edwards presents a case in *The M & M Files* where lack of documentation proved costly to an emergency physician.[8] A man found his 29-year-old wife on the floor. She was two weeks postpartum and had no medical history with the exception of migraines. She was able to walk, had no recollection of the incident, and complained that the left side of her face was numb.

On presentation to the ED, the physician noted that she had a high blood pressure of 171/110 mm Hg, was lethargic, and had a left-sided facial droop and weakness of her left upper extremity. Routine blood work, electrocardiogram, and a head CT scan were all normal. He then called the neurologist to evaluate the patient.

The patient's symptoms were resolving as the neurologist evaluated her. The ED physician recalled later that the neurologist had felt that the patient had a transient ischemic attack (TIA) and recommended that the patient be placed on aspirin and that it would be appropriate for the patient to be discharged with an outpatient work-up. The ED physician also called the patient's internist to discuss the case with him. The internist felt that the patient was having an atypical migraine and similarly could be discharged.

The patient had a seizure that night and was taken to another medical center where a second CT scan showed a cerebral infarction. Although the patient endured only minor permanent neurologic deficits, the case was reviewed. It was discovered that the dictated note of the neurologist (completed shortly after his evaluation of the patient) contained a recommendation for hospital admission. The patient's internist also retracted his recommendation concerning discharge and stated that he would have recommended admission if he had known the neurologist's recommendation (although he was convinced that it was a migraine).

continued

> The emergency physician was left without a defense because his note was brief and had no documentation of his discussions with the neurologist. It also did not contain medical reasoning as to why an outpatient evaluation was appropriate in this situation. Edwards provides the following teaching point: 'guard yourself against "memory lapses" on the part of consultants by jotting down their recommendations.'[9]

Timing of the initial and any repeated attempts at reaching the consultant becomes extremely important should the patient's condition deteriorate. Those of us who have worked in emergency rooms will all agree that there are certain consultants who are always notoriously tardy with returning phone calls. Whether it is because they are deep sleeping, lackadaisical with patient care, or just have a poor answering service, etc., these physicians pose a great liability to the ED physician if the patient's condition becomes unstable. A physician at our hospital is such a deep sleeper that the message on his answering machine instructs the caller to phone three times within one hour. If there is no response, the message requests that the police are sent to the physician's home. For this reason, most hospitals have passed by-laws requiring that consultants return phone calls from the emergency room within a reasonable time period (usually within 30 minutes). Despite this formality, ED physicians are frequently hesitant to report a colleague who is late at returning phone calls in order to maintain a good rapport with that colleague. Furthermore, it is not feasible at times for a physician to return a phone call within the required time frame (e.g. the physician may be occupied with a cardiac resuscitation, operating on a trauma patient, etc.) The lesson is that when adverse outcomes occur due to a delay in reaching a consultant, the only defense is accurate and timed documentation of attempts to reach the consultant.

The importance of using consultants to decrease the liability in your practice will be discussed in Chapter 6. We are all familiar with the emergency physicians' extensive use of consultants in their practice. However, the primary care physician should also make appropriate use of consultants. During regular office hours, you can make telephone consults to the physician of your choice or to the physician of the patient's choice. After hours, or if the first choice physician is on vacation, you can call your local ED and find out who they have on their roster call. Office consultations with specialists are helpful for medical advice, setting up follow-up appointments, or arranging for specialist evaluation and/or admission on an emergent basis. For the patient who requires an emergent disposition from the office, arranging a direct disposition with a specialist will likely save the patient hours of waiting in the emergency department. In the patient with an emergent condition, any time saved in getting the condition treated will decrease the medical liability for all of the physicians involved. The only caveat to direct arrangements of patient care from the office lies in the unstable patient. Unstable patients are best sent to the emergency department (preferably by ambulance) for immediate stabilization before admission. There should be a direct conversation between the sending physician and the receiving physician to avoid any delays.

Assessment

This is the 'glamour section' where the physician earns his or her money by coming up with the correct diagnosis. Although an accurate diagnosis is certainly the goal, there will be times when it is more important to not make an incorrect diagnosis. Even with the extensive medical training that we have all received and the superb medical technology that we have available, there are situations where we are not certain of the diagnosis. This uncertainty can lead us to either make a generalized diagnosis or commit to one (even though we are not certain).

A generalized diagnosis would be something like 'abdominal pain, unclear etiology', 'fever of unclear origin,' or 'chest pain, uncertain etiology.' In situations where a serious etiology has not been completely ruled out, we believe that a generalized diagnosis would be easier to defend in court. With a generalized diagnosis, it is more difficult for the plaintiff attorney to prove that the physician was incorrect. Physicians are less likely to be found at fault for a generalized diagnosis in their assessment. However, fault could still lie in your plan based on your assessment. In contrast, the committed (but unsure) diagnosis, is susceptible to legal scrutiny should it be found eventually to be incorrect. Think of this diagnosis as being a table with fewer legs to stand on in court than if a generalized diagnosis was used. We prefer to take the conservative approach in saying that there is minimal harm in not making a benign diagnosis, whereas there is considerable harm in making an incorrect diagnosis when a more serious one is missed.

Plan (with condition at discharge)

This section lists the treatment strategy for the patient upon cessation of your medical care for that particular visit. Always start with the disposition. Patients may be discharged home, sent to the emergency department, admitted to the hospital, etc. If the patient has a condition that requires some observation for an exacerbation after discharge (e.g. uncertain abdominal pain, gastrointestinal bleeding, febrile pediatric patient), document who they are discharged with or to. This person should be a responsible adult who can obtain medical attention for the patient. For patients sent to the emergency department for evaluation it should be noted whether they are sent by ambulance or by private vehicle. Our preference, at least with interdepartmental emergency room transfers is that they are transported by ambulance. The reason for this is the increased liability involved should the patient be involved in a motor vehicle accident or the condition worsen en route to the receiving hospital. Along with the disposition should always be the condition of the patient at discharge. This could be satisfactory, improved, or worsened. Obviously, if the condition is worsened, the patient should be discharged to a facility with a higher level of medical care.

Next, list the discharge instructions provided to the patient. The most important instructions are the signs and symptoms to seek medical care and who to follow up with. This should be included in every patient's discharge plan. Other discharge instructions could include how to take medications, what to avoid, how long to stay off work, etc. Pre-printed instructions for certain diagnoses are helpful in saving time and for ensuring details. Avoid the habit of writing 'return if symptoms worsen' or you may be hearing your patient and his or her attorney tell the court that they 'did not know what this meant.'

Finally, include the medications that you prescribe, along with any sample medications that you may distribute. Record the amount, dosage, frequency and instructions (if they can be given by more than one route). This is not only a defensive technique should there be an error in drug dispensing or administration, but also aids other health providers who may receive pharmacy calls on the patient. Remember to also include other treatments such as crutches, oxygen, Holter monitor, ultrasound prescription, etc.

References

1   Crain EF and Gershel JC (2003) *Clinical Manual of Emergency Pediatrics* (4e). McGraw-Hill, New York, New York, 698.

2   Rosen P, Barkin R *et al.* (1998) *Emergency Medicine: concepts and clinical practice* (4e). Mosby, St Louis, Missouri, 1892.

3   Bates B (1991) *A Guide to Physical Examination and History Taking* (5e). JB Lippincott, Philadelphia, Pennsylvania, 136.

4   Driscoll P, Skinner D and Earlam R (2000) *ABC of Major Trauma* (3e). BMJ Books, London, England, 94.

5   Edwards FJ (2002) *The M & M Files: morbidity and mortality rounds in emergency medicine.* Hanley & Belfus Inc., Philadelphia, Pennsylvania, 154–5.

6   Selbst SM and Korin JB (1999) *Preventing Malpractice Lawsuits in Pediatric Emergency Medicine.* American College of Emergency Physicians, Dallas, Texas, 10.

7   Pennachio DL (2004) What makes plaintiff's attorneys angry? *Medical Economics.* **81**(5): 130.

8   Edwards FJ (2002) *The M & M Files: morbidity and mortality rounds in emergency medicine.* Hanley & Belfus Inc., Philadelphia, Pennsylvania, 91–93.

9   Edwards FJ (2002) *The M & M Files: morbidity and mortality rounds in emergency medicine.* Hanley & Belfus Inc., Philadelphia, Pennsylvania, 93.

Chapter 2

Good progress note: putting it all together

- Additional chart documentation

As we have discussed in the previous chapter, there are many components to a progress note. Although it is obvious that not every patient encounter requires extensive documentation of every section, physicians should always err on the side of overdocumentation versus underdocumentation. Omit sections only when you are confident that they will have no bearing on the patient's treatment. Thorough documentation will be extremely unlikely to be detrimental to you – with the exception of the additional cost of the medical transcription and the time involved in documenting.

In contrast, poor documentation can lead to several dilemmas for you in the future. Continuing medical care may be hindered to you and other healthcare providers. Reimbursements from health plans and federal programs will be decreased. Finally, and most importantly, inadequate documentation will make your charts more susceptible to review and to scrutiny by numerous individuals. Hospitals have committees that periodically review physician notes for completeness. Similarly, managed care companies frequently examine physician notes to ensure that billing is appropriate.

Finally, a poorly documented chart is often the impetus for a plaintiff attorney to initiate a lawsuit. Lawsuits are expensive to conduct, take a long time and are extremely labor-intensive. Therefore plaintiff attorneys are selective in the cases that they choose to pursue. Indiscriminate selection of cases may lead to a heavy investment with little or no dividends (since some attorneys 'don't get paid unless you win'). One of the first items that the attorney will obtain to decide if the case is worth the endeavor will be the physician's progress note.

A clearly expressed, detailed, well thought out progress note is like a mansion with a six-foot stone fence and state-of-the-art security system protecting it. Without a doubt, you can still get sued despite good documentation, just as some thieves will still strike mansions. However, the plaintiff attorney will recognize the deterrent that a good note serves. It reminds her that you placed much thought in your medical analysis and that you are prepared to defend your actions. Remember, it is always easier to win a fight against someone who is careless and unprepared than against someone who is meticulous and on the defensive.

We hear physicians frequently complain about the time that they must set aside for documentation. Indeed, we can concur with this frustration and we, ourselves, are just as guilty. However, we must realize that we cannot change this aspect of our careers. We must not only accept it, we must do our best at it. Furthermore, expect that required or recommended documentation will most likely become more extensive in the future in order to reduce errors (e.g. Florida passed a law in July 2003 requiring that all prescriptions be printed, all dates spelled and all quantities written in both letter and number form).

The experienced and expedient physician should be able to cover each section thoroughly within the confines of a 15-minute visit most of the time. You can economize your patient interaction time by having your nurses or even the patient fill out some of the sections (e.g. allergies, medications, family history, etc.). There are also preprinted progress notes that some offices and many emergency departments use. We use a standard form for routine physical exams (i.e. school physicals, sports physicals) in the office and a standard template for the emergency department. At some hospitals, progress notes are entered on computer where medications and allergies are automatically entered into the template for the current visit. With the increased popularity of computers, this technology will become more popular and help practices become more efficient.

We cannot overly stress the importance of a thorough and detailed progress note as a vital part of defensive medicine. However, good documentation can also benefit physicians by increasing billing. It also decreases your chances of billing flaws when your charts are audited. Correct billing, as the old saying goes, determines whether a physician lives in a mansion or a cottage. Therefore, make the effort for good documentation and you will be well rewarded.

Finally, remember that a progress note may sometimes be your only source of defense in a malpractice suit. Most states have statues of limitations for initiating a malpractice lawsuit from the date of the event in question. In our state of Florida, this statute is two years. Most of us are able to reconstruct the details of a patient encounter within a couple of years from our memory and our progress note. Pediatric cases, however, are an exception that every physician should be aware of. Most states do not start the statue of limitation for malpractice claims until a pediatric patient has reached the age of 18. This means that any physician who treats children could potentially be sued 20 years from an event. Therefore, in some pediatric lawsuits, the physician has the progress note as her only source of resource. This makes it extremely difficult for the physician. It is easy for the patient and her family to remember an isolated and dramatic event while it is almost impossible for a physician to remember one out of thousands of visits (the average physician sees 5000 patient visits per year). This is particularly true if the physician is not aware of the adverse outcome and regarded the visit as a routine one. We equate this setting with the following analogy: a fight between a fighter that has been training for many years and an opponent that just discovered he is scheduled to fight and has not been training. It is not difficult to predict the side with the advantage.

There is one saving grace to these delayed pediatric cases, however. The prolonged period of involvement does make it more difficult to prove causation. This fact is highlighted by a case by Starr in *Cortlandt Forum*.[1]

Case 2.1 Time as our ally

This case involved a 58-year-old obstetrician and an eight-year-old child that he had delivered. The doctor had a very busy practice spread out across three different hospitals and included the teaching and training of obstetric residents. The child was a previously normal child who was recently diagnosed by the school psychologist as having 'learning disabilities.'

During a meeting with the child's mother, the psychologist discovered that the child had a difficult cesarean section birth filled with meconium and required resuscitation. She suggested the possibility of a link of these birth events with the child's problems. The mother decided to consult a malpractice attorney and the child's records were obtained for review. The plaintiff attorney was enthused to find from the chart that there was a significant delay from the time that the resident had notified the doctor that the baby showed signs of fetal distress to the starting time of the cesarean section. The chart documents suggested that the obstetrician was occupied with surgery at another hospital. The time that it took for him to respond to the patient in question was approximately two hours. The attorney also faulted the hospital with not finding a replacement for the obstetrician during his absence.

After obtaining an expert obstetrician's opinion to the case, the plaintiff attorney decided to proceed to trial without settlement. During the trial, the defense team argued that the child was physically normal and had no signs of hypoxic brain injury. They felt that causation of the child's learning difficulties could not be linked to an event that occurred eight years earlier and had not manifested until the psychologist's discovery. The jury felt that the plaintiff attorney did not provided enough evidence to show the delayed connection of the two events and ruled in favor of the physician. Starr writes, 'in this case, because of the tenuous link (and the intervening eight years) between the alleged negligence and the patient's subsequent difficulties in school, the jury accepted the defense lawyer's argument that the two events were unrelated and never had to decide on the physician's negligence.'[2]

Additional chart documentation

In addition to the progress note, any other professional physician–patient interaction should be documented. This includes calls from the patient, calls from the pharmacy or another healthcare provider (e.g. physical therapist, other physicians, etc.) concerning the patient, and physician calls to the patient. Documentation must contain the date and time of the interaction along with the signature of the staff member recording the interaction since they may not be the provider from the office or ED visit.

Whenever a patient calls and leaves a message for you, try to respond to the message the same day. We have witnessed many angry patients who go to the emergency department after office hours stating that they attempted to reach their physician all day and were unsuccessful. Some subsequently have emergent conditions that probably should have been treated earlier but they were waiting for their physician to call. These emergent patients represent high medical liability. Patients with non-emergent conditions may also represent increased liability because they are disgruntled. If your schedule precludes time to return patient phone calls, arrange for your colleague or a designated staff member to return the call.

Pharmacy calls should be recorded with the finest details to avoid possible medication errors. Date and time is important to include for each call. If a script is changed or cancelled, the reason should be stated in order to maintain accurate tracking of the patient's medications. This is particularly important for pain medications and antibiotics because of their potential for abuse and allergic reactions, respectively. Finally, if you call in a prescription or refill while on call, make note of it in the chart as soon as possible or you may forget.

Physician phone calls to patients are a key component to defensive medicine. First of all, patients are delighted when their physician calls them. It lets them know that their physician cared enough about their health to take the time to call. It also gives them a chance to discuss any questions that may have arisen since they last saw their physician. In addition, it gives them a sense of a stronger relationship with their physician. We have called thousands of patients during our careers and have had only one that was upset that we called. (**Case 10.21**) Reasons for physicians to call patients include giving laboratory results, checking on the patient's condition and reminding them of appointments. We will frequently call patients that we discharged with uncertain diagnoses the following day to ensure that their condition has not worsened. This technique gives you the opportunity to intervene early if their condition has worsened and is particularly useful for elderly and less educated patients who may not be able to follow your instructions well.

When a patient wants to leave before your evaluation is complete, you must decide if you are comfortable with the patient's disposition at that time. Our advice is that if there is any doubt, encourage the patient to stay for the completion of the evaluation or have the patient sign a form to leave against medical advice (AMA). This form should be included in the patient's chart and consists of four major components (in addition to the patient's name and signature, the physician's name, a witness and the date and time). The physician should complete the first three components:

1 purpose and benefit of indicated care or treatment
2 risks of refusing treatment and
3 alternative treatments.

The patient completes the final component stating why they are refusing treatment.

The purpose and benefit is usually better off written as a general statement (e.g. evaluation of chest pain). In this manner, you are not committing yourself to a diagnosis before the evaluation is complete. Stating a purpose of 'evaluation for myocardial infarction' for a patient that signs out and ultimately is found to have an aortic dissection could lead a jury to find you at fault for not telling the patient that you were evaluating her for this when she signed the form. In addition, do not use abbreviations or medical terms because it can be argued later that the patient did not understand what was written on the form. Your written language must be in laymen's terms and the patient should have an understanding of it.

The same rule applies when listing the risks of refusing treatment. Try to stay generalized, with terms like 'worsening infection', 'increase breathing difficulty', 'excessive bleeding', etc. We always include, at the end of our statement, the ultimate risk of death. We find that 'death' is one of the clearest words in the English language. Some patients have a hard time understanding anything that you tell them until they hear the word 'death.' We can imagine a plaintiff lawyer arguing for his or her deceased client's family that you were correct in all of your stated risks but never informed the patient that death could result from these risks.

The last section is for the physician to list any alternatives to the indicated treatment. If you cannot think of any reasonable alternatives, the best response would be to write 'follow up with primary physician as soon as possible with above risks.' We used to write 'none' on these forms. However, we now believe that this alternative may not be considered a true alternative to the courts. We had a patient who was in severe congestive heart failure with pulmonary edema and a potassium level of 6.8, and did not want to be hospitalized. We explained the reasons for hospitalization (i.e. cardiac monitor, treatment for pulmonary edema and hyperkalemia), the risks (i.e. lethal heart rhythm, worsening breathing status, vomiting and death) and alternatives (i.e. none). The patient signed on the form the reason for leaving was that the physician 'did not give me an alternative.' He was technically correct. We did not feel that outpatient treatment for congestive heart failure with pulmonary edema and hyperkalemia was a wise decision. In addition, 'none' should not be used, because it can sometimes be shown that there is a reasonable alternative for the patient's problem. An example is a mother who refuses an abdominal CT scan for her five-year-old child because she is concerned about the radiation and the enema contrast. A reasonable (although less accurate) alternative would be an ultrasound of the appendix. Having the mother sign the child out against medical advice because she refused a CT scan can have disastrous medical consequences for the child and for the physician legally in court.

The final point is to make sure that there is no question to future reviewers of the chart that the patient who signs out against medical advice is competent in making this decision. In particular, patients who are intoxicated with alcohol or illicit drugs, psychiatric patients, demented patients and pediatric patients represent the majority of incompetent patients. However, be alert for hypoxic patients, encephalopathic patients and head injury patients who may also be considered by the courts as incompetent in making healthcare decisions. If in doubt, treat as if the patient is incompetent or obtain the opinion of another physician.

References

1   Starr DS (2003) Medicine and the law, overextended doctor winds up in court. *Cortlandt Forum*. **16**(12): 57–9.
2   Starr DS (2003) Medicine and the law, overextended doctor winds up in court. *Cortlandt Forum*. **16**(12): 58.

Chapter 3

What you should not place in a progress note

- Conflicting data
- Prejudice or derogatory statements
- Data from other patients
- Illegible documentation
- Documentation that is not considered 'professional'

Now that we have described the essential components of the progress note, we will discuss what not to include in the progress note. Remember that any progress note has the potential to become a public document that is reviewed by many individuals. In the same manner that we treat our patients with a professional demeanor, we must treat our patient's charts with the same professionalism. Otherwise, we may become guilty of 'burning our bridges' if our own documentation is used against us in court or at deposition.

Remember that any writing in a patient's chart becomes part of the permanent record. You should not erase or alter any part of the chart documentation. You should also try to keep the documentation as objective as possible because you cannot predict who will be reading the chart in the future. These potential chart readers may not understand the context in which the writer made his inputs. Therefore, the following are things that should be considered sacred to progress notes.

Conflicting data

In general, data that are placed in a progress note should not be conflicting. It is well known that a fight is easier to win when the other side is fighting among themselves. Indeed, you can be sure that a plaintiff attorney will use any contradictory information or arguments in the patient's chart against the defending physician(s). In fact, he may even use your own staff or colleagues to testify against you. This almost certain embarrassment is usually avoidable by reading your charts and avoiding contradictory information.

What are examples of conflicting data? The most common one is discrepancy in findings between nurse and doctor. As we discussed previously, it is prudent to read all the entries in the chart for the patient on the day of the visit. This will optimize the care that the patient receives because it encompasses the observations of multiple healthcare employees. In addition, if you find a difference between your findings and that of a nurse, you and the nurse can try to ascertain why the difference exists before recording your findings on the chart.

Another example would be differences among physicians. An important distinction needs to be made in these instances. Differences in opinions (i.e. treatment plans, differential diagnoses) are not uncommon among physicians and do not necessarily reflect conflicting data. These data are partly subjective and differences could exist. In contrast, medical exam findings (e.g. heart murmur, respiratory wheezes) and diagnostic test interpretations (e.g. electrocardiogram, chest X-ray) are usually more objective (but not always) and are less subject to reviewer differences. These discrepancies often serve as fuel and ammunition for plaintiff attorneys. Therefore, if they must exist in your chart, try to explain why and always maintain a diplomatic tone in the chart.

Finally, differences may occur in objective data such as vital signs and laboratory data. Although these differences are sometimes accurate and reflect changes in the patient's condition, more frequently they represent error in technique or equipment (e.g. improper blood pressure cuff, blood from another patient).

Case 3.1 Do we have the right sample?

We treated a patient who presented with chest pain. The patient had a non-diagnostic EKG but his blood had been mislabeled with another patient's name. The cardiac enzymes were reported as very elevated, suggesting myocardial damage. He was treated in the hospital for acute myocardial infarction for 24 hours before the mistake was discovered. The patient from which the blood results were from had a diagnostic EKG and was taken to the cardiac catheterization laboratory. No significant harm occurred to either patient involved but there certainly could have been severe consequences. Mistakes in error or equipment are inevitable (*see* Chapter 8) but should be minimized. Plaintiff attorneys will utilize them in their cases.

Inevitably, there will be times when conflicting data will be in the chart. During these times, it is important to remain diplomatic and avoid connotations that may sound condescending, disapproving, arrogant, or omniscient. Consider thoroughly why there are data that is different from yours. This way, you not only keep an open-mind to other possibilities in the medical evaluation, but you also mentally prepare yourself to defend yourself in court in the event that you are asked to do so.

Prejudice or derogatory statements

Prejudices and biases are best left to private conversations (or not said at all) and definitely should not be in a legal document. Statements of this nature are not only non-professional but show disrespect for the patient. Showing disrespect for a patient in the progress note is unjustifiable and will serve no other purpose than to degrade the reputation of the guilty physician (regardless of whether the comments are true or false).

As physicians, we were taught and trained to be professionals. We will all probably be involved in arguments and discrepancies with patients at some point in our careers. Likewise, we will find that some patients will get 'under our skin' at some point. However, professionalism entails that we weather these dilemmas without subjective criticism in the chart. Remember that others who may read your chart may not share the same opinion as you and that the patient does not have the opportunity to defend himself from these comments. These issues will definitely come into consideration by lawyers and judges should your note be submitted for trial. As Roediger and Salmon memorably wrote: 'think twice about what you write – it could later become Exhibit 1 in a case against you.'[1] A colleague of ours admitted an alcoholic patient while on an unassigned call. In his progress note, he wrote that the patient 'will continue to be a menace to society upon discharge.' Although this statement could very likely be true, it is easy to see how inappropriate and damaging physician comments can be (e.g. What will the opinions of future physicians who read this note be even before they treat the patient?).

We have also been told stories of emergency physicians in the past referring to unpleasant patients in the chart as 'GOMERs.' This is an acronym for 'Get Out of My ER.' However, we do not see the term used anymore and only hear it mentioned among healthcare staff from time to time. This is a positive aspect of medicine that the current legal environment has fostered.

Data from other patients

The above statement sounds simple and easy to follow. The misplacement of data and labs is not an uncommon occurrence. There are multiple reasons outside of natural human error why this happens. In a crowded and busy emergency department or office, patients get moved from one examination room to another frequently. For example, a patient may need the specific equipment in a trauma room or a gynecologic room in order to be appropriately examined. In addition, some patients are moved out into hall beds after they have been examined. In the process of playing 'musical patients,' a patient's file is often left in the previous chart; or the doctor or nurse may not be aware that the patient has been relocated. It then becomes easy to misplace information in the same manner that mail becomes misplaced when a person changes address.

Another example takes place when data is obtained without labeling the patient from which the data was obtained. Trauma patients will sometimes come in as 'John Doe' and have blood drawn, EKG performed, etc. that are all unlabeled or labeled as John Doe. After their identity is discovered, there may be data with two different names pertaining to the same individual. The chest pain patient will also typically receive an immediate electrocardiogram upon entering the emergency department even before his name is obtained. Due to the voluminous paperwork that is present in most clinical practices, any piece of paper that does not have an identifying name has the potential to be lost or misplaced. Edwards writes in *The M & M Files*, 'when faced with a desk full of lab reports, charts, and EKGs – it is only a matter of time before Murphy's law asserts itself, unless scrupulous care is taken to match names to studies.'[2]

Finally, patients often have the same or similar names. Most hospitals have created 'name alert' warnings to keep medical staff aware but the potential for confusion is never eliminated. Name confusion is a problem that plagues every business and profession. Physicians should make a habit of noting a patient's name before they examine them. Patients should not be regarded as 'room nine' or 'the abdominal pain.'

Case 3.2 Always look at the name

In *The M & M Files*, Edwards presents a case of how an identification error leads to a disastrous and fatal result.[3] A 51-year-old man came to the ED with an episode of left shoulder discomfort and 'chest weakness' that had started a few hours prior to his visit and had subsided. The patient noted that he was stressed and depressed over losing his job recently and only came in because his wife had insisted. His cardiac risk factors included 'mild' hypertension, tobacco use until one year ago, and a father that had a myocardial infarction in his later years.

The patient had a normal physical examination. His chest X-ray, EKG, and cardiac enzymes were also normal. After a stay of three hours in the department, he had no recurrence of the pain and wanted to go home. The emergency physician discharged him with a prescription of alprazolam to help his sleep and instructed him to follow up with his primary physician as soon as possible.

The following morning, the patient went into full cardiac arrest and was not able to be resuscitated in the ED. Severe coronary artery disease with signs of an acute myocardial infarction was shown on his autopsy. When the case was reviewed, there were two EKGs found in the patient's chart. The normal EKG that the ED physician had seen during the initial visit belonged to another patient. The other patient's name was clearly written on it. The deceased patient's EKG, however, had unequivocal ST segment elevation in leads V4-V6. 'A lawsuit was subsequently settled on behalf of the patient's estate.'[2]

Illegible documentation

Illegible handwriting has always been a complaint against physicians. We have often heard people make jokes like 'he can't write neat, he is a physician' or 'his handwriting is terrible, he must be hiding something.' Although there may be reasons for our handwriting to appear sloppy such as writing too fast or using too many shorthand notations, we do not believe that poor handwriting has a direct association with our profession. There are plenty of lawyers, teachers, law officers, etc. (you name the profession) who have handwriting that is difficult to read. We believe that the reason that physicians receive more criticism than other professionals is the enormous amount of spontaneous writing that we must do. Most of the writing that we do (e.g. prescriptions, hospital progress notes, emergency room notes, consultations, etc.) needs to be done in a timely fashion in order to deliver immediate information. We frequently do not have the convenience of a transcriptionist available for our immediate needs. In addition, the notes that we write have substantial roles in the healthcare of our patients. Therefore, handwritten physician notes are subjected to more review and criticism than those of other professions. As the author Inga Dubay stated, 'it isn't that their handwriting is any worse than anyone else's. It's just that theirs really counts. It can be a matter of life or death.'[4]

The statements in the previous paragraph are in no means an excuse for illegible documentation. They are made to emphasize the importance of writing legibly. An easy-to-read note may take the physician a bit longer to write, but will save the physician time in the long run. Nurses will be able to give discharge instructions and carry out orders without confirming with the physician. Secretaries will not check with the physician as to the diagnosis and follow-up appointment. Finally, clarification calls from the pharmacies will be minimized.

A special mention is fitting here concerning illegible medication orders. A recent study by the Agency for Healthcare Research and Quality showed that approximately 6% of United States hospital patients injured by medication errors are a result of poor handwriting. These injuries account for 777 000 patients and cost $1.5 to $5.6 billion dollars each year.[4]

Case 3.3 The pen can be deadly

The classic example that has appeared in numerous publications is that of a Texas cardiologist who was found liable for a patient who died after being given a wrong medication.[5] The physician had written for 20mg of Isordil but was given 20mg of Plendil (twice the maximum daily dose) by the pharmacist. In our home state of Florida, legislators recently took extra measures in reducing prescription errors by mandating that all prescriptions be typed or handwritten, have the date written out, and have the quantity dispensed written out in full in addition to the numerical value. Helpful habits include placing a zero in front of all decimal points, writing out the word 'units' ('u' can be mistaken for a zero or a four), and being aware of drugs with similar names (e.g. Zoloft or Zocor, Ceftin or Cefzil, Celebrex or Cerebyx).[5]

In addition, notes that are clear and legible will be impressive to other professionals. Consultants and other healthcare providers will enjoy a productive working relationship with you if they are able to read your notes. In contrast, if your notes are illegible, they will be forced to spend more time interpreting it. They will also be increasing their liability due to the greater potential for error from misinterpretation. Unambiguous handwriting will also create an impression to lawyers and judges that the physician has 'nothing to hide' and is meticulous in his work. (Whether this is true or not depends on the particular physician.)

Documentation that is not considered 'professional'

A patient's chart is a legal document that can be subjected to legal review. Hence, its contents should always look as professional as possible. A professional-appearing chart makes the physician appear competent and meticulous. In contrast, an unprofessional-appearing chart makes the physician appear careless and sloppy.

The consensus with the professionals that we have worked with through the years is that only black or blue ink pens are acceptable. Red ink and pencil (two others that are commonly used) are definitely not acceptable. Avoid inks that tend to smear because you may end up with a dirty-looking progress note.

Avoid cramming information in order to get all of your information into one sheet. This not only makes everything look messy, but you may not be able to read it yourself years later when you have forgotten the incident. Do not use paper that is not appropriately labeled with office or hospital overhead (i.e. notebook paper). It is acceptable to submit a patient-generated medical sheet on notebook paper.

Finally, your progress note is essentially an extension of your appearance. It has to look clean, meticulous, and professional in the same manner that you do. We cannot recall a specific case from our readings or our experiences that was lost specifically because of a 'bad' chart; however, a professionally kept chart gives the physician a positive image.

References

1   Roediger J and Salmon PM (2003) Making changes in charts? *Physicians Practice*. **13**(6): 65.*

2   Edwards FJ (2002) *The M & M Files: morbidity and mortality rounds in emergency medicine*. Hanley & Belfus Inc., Philadelphia, Pennsylvania, 67.

3   Edwards FJ (2002) *The M & M Files: morbidity and mortality rounds in emergency medicine*. Hanley & Belfus Inc., Philadelphia, Pennsylvania, 66–7.

4   Greene L (2003) Clearly curing the confusion. *St Petersburg Times*. **August 2**: 7A.

5   Adams D (2003) Florida tells doctors: Print clearly or else. *American Medical News*. **46**(29): 4.

Chapter 4

Things to avoid doing clinically

- Avoid treating problems that you have never treated before
- Avoid giving the diagnosis of constipation (most of the time)
- Avoid letting your patient or others influence your medical recommendations
- Avoid accepting a patient's history if there is conflicting data from others
- Avoid ignoring abnormal vital signs
- Avoid ignoring nurses' comments
- Avoid ignoring your patient's concerns
- Avoid assumptions and avoid giving diagnoses when you are unsure
- Avoid the belief that 'gold standards' are golden
- Avoid treating children in the same manner as adults

Avoid treating problems that you have never treated before

Clinical problems that a physician has never treated before or has had very little experience with treating are usually best to defer to a more experienced physician. The physician should remember that clinical practice is not similar to residency training where you frequently receive praise and accommodation for taking on a new challenge. In contrast, the practicing physician is expected (as she should be) by the public to be an expert who can make decisions confidently. There is a small margin for error in actual practice and the consequences of failure can be severe. One of the favorite questions asked by plaintiff attorneys during deposition is, 'Doctor, can you please tell me how many times in your career you have treated this particular problem?' It is easy to see how devastating the response to this question can be to the physician's defense. With reference to a family physician treating a problem that he has never treated before and is later sued for, Starr in his *Cortlandt Forum* column 'Medicine and the Law' writes, 'perhaps he would have been better off referring the patient to a specialty clinic. This model is followed by many competent and independent family physicians across the country.'[1] As an alternative, if the physician has the strong desire to treat the problem, she can improve her legal position if she discusses the problem with a consultant who is knowledgeable with it. Any conversation must, of course, be well documented in the chart.

Be careful with problems or procedures that you have not encountered frequently or have not done in a long time. Plaintiff attorneys frequently ask (and will look for confirmation) how many times you have treated a certain problem or performed a particular procedure. Furthermore, they will follow up these questions with asking when you last treated the problem or performed the procedure. Therefore, providing medical care that is not routine for your practice not only constitutes increased legal liability but also creates increased medical liability because your skills and knowledge may not be as sharp as they once were or should be.

Case 4.1 Recognizing one's limitations

Starr provides an example in the *Cortlandt Forum* journal.[2] This case involved a cardiothoracic surgeon who mainly treated adults but occasionally would perform 'simple' pediatric operations. Despite having not performed surgery for a patent ductus arteriosus (PDA) in five years, the surgeon decided to perform the surgery on a 26-week premature baby. This was an elective procedure that the surgeon had chosen to do. He opted not to defer the procedure to more experienced cardiac surgeons at another hospital.

The surgery was a disaster as the surgeon not only could not find the patent ductus but he also damaged the phrenic nerve during the surgery. The baby had a complicated post-operative course on the ventilator and developed severe damage to her lungs and brain. A lawsuit was filed against the surgeon. The case went to trial five years later. Although the defense made valid arguments that the patient's lung and brain damage were a consequence of her premature birth, these arguments were to no avail. 'The jury's decision was not based on the technical testimony of the experts but on their anger toward a physician who had performed a procedure outside of his training and experience, with disastrous results.'[3]

Avoid giving the diagnosis of constipation (most of the time)

This is especially true in the emergency setting but also applies in the primary care setting. The temptation, however, is there because: 'constipation is the most common digestive complaint in the United States and accounts for 2.5 million physician visits per year.'[4] Unless the patient is young, healthy, has had no abdominal surgeries, has a benign abdominal exam, has normal vital signs, and has a prior history of constipation, you should be skeptical about diagnosing constipation without further tests. Stark writes, 'note that recent onset of constipation without any historical basis may suggest mechanical obstructive causes.'[5] We have found much truth in this statement in our practice. We have seen two patients that were treated by their primary physicians for constipation and given stool softeners, laxatives, and enemas over two to three days without improvement and with no other medical evaluation. One turned out to have a small bowel obstruction and the other had diverticulitis with a bowel perforation and an abscess.

Case 4.2 Not as simple as it sounds

Another case involved a 21-year-old male who was seen at a walk-in-clinic for abdominal pain and treated for constipation with enemas. He presented to our ED four hours later and had a tender right lower quadrant on abdominal exam and was subsequently found to have acute appendicitis on CT scan. This dogma is particularly true in the emergency setting. Our colleague from Jacksonville Emergency Consultants, Jorge Perez-Povada, MD told us once, 'giving the diagnosis of constipation in the emergency department will eventually land you a lawsuit.' Remember, missing the diagnosis of constipation is probably not going to result in any harm. In contrast, accepting the diagnosis of constipation without considering serious causes of obstipation can lead to detrimental therapeutics for the patient.

Case 4.3 Simple diagnoses may have serious causes

Edwards presents a case, in *The M & M Files*, where the physician accepted the diagnosis of constipation with grave consequences.[6] A 55-year-old woman, who did not speak any English, presented to the ED by ambulance complaining of abdominal pain. The triage nurse obtained a limited history from the patient's son, who had a very limited English vocabulary.

The patient complained of abdominal pain and constipation. She had not had a bowel movement for four days and was taking Tylenol with codeine and ibuprofen for the pain. The son also reported that the patient had a history of peptic ulcer disease in the distant past. Her vital signs on initial presentation were unremarkable and her physical exam revealed: 'normal bowel sounds, and nonspecific tenderness in lower quadrants more than upper.'[7] There was no guarding or rebound of the abdomen. Her stool was hemoccult negative.

An X-ray of the abdomen showed an abundance of stool while there were some abnormalities on the patient's blood work. The potassium and bicarbonate were slightly low at 3.1 mEq/L and 16 mEq/L, respectively. The white blood cell count was normal but there was a left shift with 18% band forms. The patient's pain seemed to worsen after she was given oral fluids, a bottle of magnesium citrate, and a soap suds enema. She was then given an injection of 60 mg of ketorolac for the pain. Shortly afterwards, the patient had a bowel movement and the ED physician wrote up her discharge against the wishes of the patient's son.

Before the patient was discharged, she quickly became unresponsive and hypotensive with a systolic blood pressure less than 50 mm Hg. She was intubated and resuscitated with fluids and dopamine. The subsequent chest X-ray revealed subdiaphragmatic free air from a presumed perforated viscus. The patient expired in the intensive care unit the following day. The autopsy showed a perforation of a duodenal ulcer, signs of a small bowel

continued

obstruction, and frank pus in the peritoneal cavity. The family complained to hospital administration about how the patient was felt to be eligible for discharge.

The ED physician in this case had a preconceived diagnosis of his patient's problem based on the patient's limited history. He did not become alarmed when some of the patient's laboratory values were abnormal. Constipation should never be accepted as the diagnosis when there is evidence of a metabolic acidosis or there is evidence of a left shift on the complete blood count. These suggest either a severe bacterial infection, a severe stressor to the normal physiologic state, or both. He also was adamant against abandoning his preconception both when the patient's pain became worse in the ED and when the patient's son felt that she was not well enough to be discharged. Remember that the diagnosis of constipation is one of exclusion and one that a physician better be pretty darn sure of.

Avoid letting your patient or others influence your medical recommendations

Patients and their family members will often try to convince physicians to alter their treatment recommendations. They may do this for several reasons including: convenience, financial, cultural, etc. Some patients may not want to be admitted or may not want to return the next day for a re-evaluation based on their prior commitments. Some patients will ask for cheaper substitute medications because they cannot afford the ones that you recommend. Finally, some may have cultural beliefs against certain medical treatments such as parents who do not believe in immunizations for their children.

These situations can become liability traps if the physician is not careful. Alternating treatment regimens to satisfy a patient may lead to suboptimal or inadequate treatment or follow-up. These consequences result in the increased probability of an unfavorable outcome. In the event of an adverse outcome, a liability suit may be difficult to defend due to substandard medical care or poor documentation of the patient's desire for an alternative treatment plan.

Physicians should listen to their patient's (and their family's) requests. At times, they may actually be reasonable and comparable to the physician's own plan. If this is the case, allowing the patient to follow his own plan will certainly increase the likelihood of compliance. The majority of the time, however, the patient's plan will entail some compromise of the physician's plan. The physician must then decide whether there is an increase in the potential for treatment failure. If there is, the physician must adamantly adhere to his plan. If the risk is only minor, the physician can consider following the patient's plan but adhere to it only after he thoroughly documents several things. The physician should clearly state why his plan was recommended, why the patient wanted his plan, and the risks that are involved by not following the recommended plan.

Case 4.4 Sticking with one's gut instinct

Starr presents a case in *Corlandt Forum* where a patient did not follow his doctor's recommendation and suffered an adverse outcome.[8] The case involved a family practitioner with an expertise in diabetic management and a 54-year-old man with type II diabetes who had a foot wound. The patient visited the physician complaining of redness and swelling in his foot. After the physician examined the patient's foot, he opened a blister and drained purulent material from it. Afterwards, he wanted to admit the patient to the hospital for further wound care. The patient, however, pleaded with him to not do so because it was around Christmas time and he had bills to pay. The physician obliged and sent the patient home on oral antibiotics and told him to return for follow-up in one week (giving him enough time to handle his business).

A couple of nights later, the pain grew worse and the patient came to the emergency department. He was diagnosed with a 'deep infection of the foot' and admitted for intravenous antibiotics. He also required intravenous insulin to treat his blood sugar, which was greater than 500 mg/dl. The infection was difficult to treat and the patient had half of his foot amputated the following week. After extensive rehabilitation, the patient was finally able to walk again without pain. He subsequently filed a malpractice suit against his family practitioner.

On review of the physician's progress note, it was written that there was 'the presence of a painful blister with local redness and an infected tract along a medial tendon.'[9] This statement was very damaging to the physician's case. We are all aware that infections in diabetics can be difficult to treat. Moreover, most of us would consider only simple and uncomplicated skin infections as ones that are candidates for outpatient therapy. The statement above suggested that the infection may have spread to the deeper tissues and would not be considered simple. Furthermore, diabetic infections should usually be rechecked in a shorter time frame than a week.

The physician also damaged his case by not checking a blood sugar during the office visit. This test is so inexpensive, quick, and easy that it is almost routinely performed in diabetics, particularly in diabetics with infections. Even if the patient cannot afford the test, you would probably gain more by doing it, documenting the result, and writing off the cost. It is not uncommon for infections to trigger off diabetic ketoacidosis events. Furthermore, an uncontrolled blood sugar suggests that a more conservative treatment regimen is warranted to ensure proper healing. Peripheral vascular disease, non-compliance, and peripheral neuropathy are all associated with uncontrolled blood sugar and non-healing wounds.

Indeed, the plaintiff expert endocrinologist took advantage of the issues discussed in the preceding paragraph. He stated that the physician should either have immediately admitted the patient for intravenous antibiotics, or alternatively, have had the patient return the following day for a repeat

continued

evaluation. He was also critical of the fact that the patient's extremely elevated blood sugar was not discovered earlier. The expert felt that it contributed to the worsening of the infection. We agree with this statement and offer this analogy. Bacteria are difficult to treat if you are trying to kill them (with antibiotics) and you are feeding them (with sugar) at the same time. The patient also helped his case when the jury witnessed his hobbling around the courtroom. The jury found in favor of the patient and awarded him $1.5 million.

Although it is debatable if the outcome would have been different if the patient had been immediately admitted for intravenous antibiotics, it was enough for the plaintiff attorney to show that there was deviation from the standard of care and that this contributed to the patient's injuries. Furthermore, the physician was not given consideration for attempting to comply with his patient's wishes. Starr writes that 'such factors are rarely considered by the jury in reducing the blame assigned to the physician.'[10] A short note in the patient's chart can be used to draw the jury's consideration (e.g. 'recommend inpatient treatment but patient requests outpatient treatment').

Avoid accepting a patient's history if there is conflicting data from others

The patients that are often guilty of this include elderly demented patients, young children, intoxicated patients, and psychiatric patients. Of course there is also the patient that will intentionally give you a false history for secondary gain (e.g. worker's compensation) or to avoid punishment (e.g. illicit drug user). As a physician, you are a detective and must assimilate all of the evidence and decide what will be useful in your evaluation.

Case 4.5 Who should one believe?

On separate occasions, we have seen two elderly, mildly demented patients because caregivers at their nursing homes had seen them with difficulty swallowing their food. Both patients presented in no acute distress and stated that they felt fine. They also denied any difficulty ingesting their food. We did barium swallow studies in both patients. One had a large piece of meat lodged in her proximal esophagus, while the other had complete obstruction of her mid-esophagus.

Avoid ignoring abnormal vital signs

Vital signs are the most objective section of the progress note outside of the patient's demographics. They are not subjected to human skill or bias when they are performed correctly. Therefore, the jury and the judge will have no other conclusion for abnormal vital signs than an underlying medical condition.

Furthermore, plaintiff attorneys have extensive references of normal and abnormal vital signs. During the trial, they will probably magnify these references by 10 and ask the physician to explain why an abnormal vital sign was not addressed.

Ideally, vital signs should be taken prior to the physician–patient interaction. This enables the physician to create a mental picture of the patient's illness and also to be ready to address any abnormality. Patients are typically not charged for repeat vital signs, so repeat as often as necessary. They should definitely be repeated after any therapeutic intervention, medicine administration, or prolonged observation. Although the physician will not be able to correct or explain all abnormal vital signs during a visit, the goal should be to rule out serious causes, document stability of the abnormal vital signs, give the patient instructions to avoid worsening of the problem (e.g. avoid decongestants for increased blood pressure, caffeine for tachycardia), and assure close follow-up.

We have reviewed a few cases where sepsis was missed on the initial visit to the emergency department. In most of these cases, the patients did not appear in any distress. Their white blood cell counts were minimally elevated. Their vital signs, however, were abnormal. Specifically, one patient had a blood pressure of 90/70 mm Hg and a pulse of 108 beats/minute. Another patient had a temperature of 103°F with other vital signs being normal. The final patient had a pulse of 125 beats/minute and the remaining vitals were within the normal range. All three patients were admitted on return visits with complicated sepsis. When the lawsuits were filed in these cases, the primary argument was that these patients were discharged in the presence of vital signs that suggested sepsis. Although these were not our patients, we were familiar with their cases. None of the patients appeared toxic on their initial presentation. Their abnormal vital signs could have been regarded as nonspecific findings. However, to a plaintiff attorney who has a medical textbook describing the changes in the vital signs with sepsis, these numbers are concrete evidence that a diagnosis was missed.

Avoid ignoring nurses' comments

Nurses, like physicians, want to know what is bothering the patients that they take care of. They will often get their own history from the patient and perform their own examination and document these findings on the chart. While most physicians will agree that an experienced nurse's comments and findings are often helpful, there will be times when their findings will be different than yours. In these situations, it is helpful to acknowledge that you are aware of the nurse's findings but cannot confirm them at this time. In this manner, the statements in the chart are not conflicting and subjected to future debate. Physicians appear arrogant when they ignore nurses' comments. Their evaluation is also considered incomplete if they do not consider the nurse's comments.

Whenever the nurse's findings differ from the physician's findings, the physician should discuss these 'nursing' findings with that particular nurse to determine if they could be legitimate. The physician should be fairly receptive to take merit in the nurse's findings even if the finding is not apparent to the physician. Remember that a patient's history and/or condition can change between evaluations and the nurse is a trained healthcare professional. In addition, nurses will probably spend more time with the patient than the physician.

Case 4.6 A nurse's intuition

A clinical example came with one of our nurses. A 23-year-old female with a six-month pregnancy presented to our emergency department with nausea and vomiting. She stated that these symptoms had been present for three months and that she had been to another emergency department six times. We evaluated her extensively with blood tests, urinalysis, and gall-bladder ultrasound, all of which were unremarkable. Since we did not see her throw up during her stay in the ED, we had written up her discharge. Her nurse asked us to order a urine drug screen. The nurse had taken care of her and developed a clinical suspicion. The drug screen was positive for marijuana and phencyclidine. The patient was reported to the Department of Children and Families for unborn child abuse.

Avoid ignoring your patient's concerns

The physician should listen to the patient's medical concerns whether they are legitimate or not. Listening to a patient is a time-honored tradition and leads to a good physician–patient relationship. In addition, it lets the patient (and others who review the chart) know that the physician cared about him. Remember that patients are less likely to sue and lawyers are less likely to win suits if the physician showed that he was receptive and caring. In contrast, patients will become angry if they are not heard. Jurors will perceive the physician as arrogant and unsympathetic if they do not listen to their patients.

Case 4.7 Another case of 'my doctor did not listen to me'

Starr presents a case in *Cortlandt Forum* where a large amount was awarded, partly because the physician appeared uncaring to his patient's concerns.[11] A 28-year-old woman had a difficult delivery of a 7 lb 10 oz boy that was complicated by pelvic outlet obstruction and shoulder dystocia. The boy had no permanent complications. One year later, she was under the care of a different obstetrician for her second pregnancy.

During a third trimester visit, an ultrasound examination estimated the birth weight at 9.5 lb. The patient responded to this news from her physician by saying that she hoped 'the baby wouldn't have the same problems as my first one.' There was no apparent response of the physician to this remark. On a visit four days after her due date, the patient testified that she had questioned her physician again about the potential of problems with the size of this baby. Again, she felt that her concern was ignored.

When the patient went into labor the following day, the second baby's

---

continued

shoulder was also caught on the pelvic outlet. The obstetrician had to use a vacuum extractor along with strenuous effort to deliver the baby. The traumatic delivery resulted in a severe injury to the child's brachial plexus. The injury's severity required several corrective surgeries over the next few years. The patient was predicted to never gain full function of his arm. He was also likely to develop chronic pain and scoliosis of the spine.

The main basis of the plaintiff's argument was that the physician did not take notice of her prior difficult delivery. In failing to do so, he also did not properly anticipate or prepare for the problems that arose during her second delivery. Starr writes that 'brushing aside her worries looked extremely indifferent at trial.'[12] It also allowed the lawyer to exclaim, 'if only the doctor had listened.'[12] The award was for $13.3 million to the plaintiff after the jury was allowed to see the four-year-old boy and listen to the handicaps that he would face throughout his life.

Avoid assumptions and giving diagnoses when you are unsure

Although the public may feel that we have all of the medical answers when they come to see us, we all know that this misconception is far from true. There will often be times when our evaluation helps us eliminate some possible causes but does not allow us to reach any definite cause. We have told hundreds of patients through the years that we are unsure of what is causing their problem. We cannot remember an instance where a reasonable patient has become upset at us for telling them this. Most of the time, they are appreciative of the effort that we gave in their evaluation and our sincerity and honesty with them. We have had some psychosocial patients that have non-organic medical problems who have become upset at not getting a definitive diagnosis. They will utter comments like 'five hours in the emergency room for you to tell me that!' or 'all of those tests and you do not have an answer!' This does not bother us because, as we mentioned before, it is better to say that you are unsure then to give an incorrect diagnosis.

As previously mentioned, it is always better to confirm medical data if possible. Assumptions can sometimes be made based on false pretenses, personal biases, or incomplete evaluation. Remember that assumptions are difficult to defend to the plaintiff lawyers, judge, jury, or even your own defense attorney. There is a famous wise adage, 'when you assume, you make an (ass) of you (u) and (me).'

Case 4.8 Getting one's foot out of one's mouth

Starr, in an article from *Cortlandt Forum*, writes about a particular case that we feel highlights the above adage.[13] The case involves a well-respected family physician who had developed a reputation as a local tuberculosis (TB) expert because he had extensive experience in treating TB in the area.

continued

Other physicians frequently referred TB patients to him. The doctor was presented a patient with allergy symptoms, chronic cough, and night sweats. He ordered a chest X-ray and read it as 'a suspicious fibrotic mass with possible cavitation in the upper lung.'

The physician informed the patient that he probably had TB and began treating him with a dual drug regimen and home quarantine, and informed him that he must inform his contacts. The patient complied with the treatment regimen for one year but his symptoms did not get better and his chest X-ray went unchanged. The patient obtained a second opinion from a pulmonologist. The second physician ordered another X-ray which was interpreted as 'old, inactive scarring, possibly histoplasmosis.' Tuberculosis cultures were ordered and were subsequently negative.

The patient subsequently sued the initial physician for 'emotional damage', side effects of medications, and lost wages from being quarantined. Not surprisingly, the family practitioner lost the case because his defense was weakened because of the one (although huge) assumption that he had made (i.e. he assumed that all upper lung cavitation was TB). We have read about similar assumptions and lawsuits concerning physicians making the diagnosis of HIV based on CD4 counts and not obtaining HIV tests.

Case 4.9 Look beyond the obvious

Levine described in *Medical Economics* another case of assumption that almost led to a disastrous outcome.[14] During a call night of her senior year of an internal medicine residency, she was called to admit a patient from the emergency department. The patient had a history of metastatic prostate cancer and was brought in unresponsive. The ED physician felt that the patient had just suffered a big stroke, which caused his unresponsiveness. Since his family did not want any aggressive treatment due to his terminal condition, the resident was asked to admit the patient so his family could see him for the last time.

After seeing the patient, the resident did not disagree with the ED physician's plan and wrote orders for the patient to be taken to a floor bed. Although the ED nurse questioned the sense of sending off blood work, the resident requested a complete blood count, serum electrolytes, and serum glucose. As the patient was being transported to the floor, the patient's daughter was able to give some history leading up to the unresponsiveness. She said that her father had been doing well and had some sugars that were high recently. His doctor, therefore, started him on some pills for this. The resident did not take alarm of this history.

Shortly later, the resident checked the computer for labs results but they were still pending. She then went to sleep and did not wake up in time to recheck them before the morning rounds. Her attending physician called her at 11 am and informed her that the patient's blood sugar was 10 mg/dl. After she gave a stat order to infuse dextrose intravenously, the patient

continued

woke up and had a normal neurologic exam. She was informed by another physician five years later that the patient was still doing fine. This case is a fine example to not assume that the evaluation of another physician is correct when there is evidence to suggest otherwise.

Case 4.10 Avoiding prejudices from prior experiences

Edwards presents a case, in *The M & M Files*, where an assumption led to an insult and an incorrect diagnosis.[15] A 76-year-old lady was brought to the ED after she had fallen on her left shoulder. The patient did not know why she had fallen but her daughter brought up some additional concerns to the ED physician. She noted that her mother was extremely active three months ago and could drive herself several hundred miles without any problems. Lately, however, she had become forgetful, untidy, and had poor balance.

The ED physician noted a stench of alcohol in the room and believed that this patient was a 'closet alcoholic' because he had seen a similar case a few days earlier. He asked the patient several times during the physical examination about her alcohol consumption because the patient in the next cubicle was extremely noisy. She told him that she had an occasional glass of brandy and still had half of the bottle that her daughter gave her five years ago. The physician did not believe her story and questioned the daughter about her mother's alcohol intake.

The physical exam was unremarkable with the exception of several bruises. The physician ordered an X-ray of the shoulder. There was no fracture seen and the physician discharged the patient. He informed her to follow up with her own physician as soon as possible. He felt that the patient's physician should perform the work-up for these additional concerns. The patient was not able to get an appointment with her own physician for two weeks.

Several days after the ED visit, the patient fell again. The daughter decided to take her to another ED where a different physician performed a thorough neurologic exam and discovered a pronator drift and several other abnormalities. A subsequent CT of the head showed a large brain tumor. The daughter filed a complaint against the first ED physician for the missed diagnosis. She was also upset at the physician's assumption that her mother's problems were from alcohol abuse. The complaint led to a review of the case. It was discovered that the alcohol stench was not from the patient in question but was from the noisy patient in the next cubicle.

The initial ED physician made two ill-advised assumptions in this case. He assumed that the alcohol smell in the room belonged to the patient. It did not matter to him that this assumption was not supported from the responses of the patient or those of her daughter. If he had felt strongly that alcohol was the problem, it was his burden to prove this by ordering a blood alcohol level. The second assumption is that this lady's fall was due to a benign etiology. There were many red flags in this case and a work-up for syncope should have been instigated.

Avoid the belief that 'gold standards' are golden

We have developed certain tests in medicine that are called 'gold standards.' This designation is given mainly because they are the best available tests for certain medical conditions. Unfortunately, some physicians falsely believe that they are 'perfect' tests and have 100% sensitivity. Besides the inherent limitations of these tests themselves, they are also subjected to the element of human error.

A typical example is that of the cardiac catheterization. Currently, this is the test of choice for the detection of coronary artery disease. A patient with a completely normal catheterization is usually referred 'for evaluation of non-cardiac chest pain.' In turn, many ED physicians will base their disposition decisions based on these negative catheterization reports. This practice, which is relatively within the 'standard of care', is not free from error. We have seen a few cases of myocardial infarctions from coronary spasms from patients with 'clean' coronaries. In addition, we have seen patients with 'normal' catheterizations who have repeat catheterizations showing significant coronary artery disease within the same year. This suggests that human error is also present in these procedures.

Case 4.11 Test is only as good as its interpreter

The next example is from our vascular surgery colleague, James Balliro, MD. A few years ago, he was consulted to review a carotid angiogram on a patient with stroke symptoms. The patient had a carotid angiogram, the 'gold standard' for evaluation of the carotid arteries. The test was read as normal by two separate radiologists. However, the patient was still having stroke symptoms. Therefore, our colleague was consulted to review the study. He was surprised to see that a carotid dissection was present on the study. As the patient was being prepared for surgery, the dissection extended and the patient expired. The delay in surgery was in part due to the admitting physician's reliance on the gold standard interpretation by the radiologist. Is a test still the best test if it is read incorrectly?

The second point about 'gold standards' is that they are sometimes not practical and increase our legal risks. For example, during our combined 18 years of practicing medicine, we rarely see a pulmonary angiogram, or a venogram ordered for evaluation of pulmonary embolus and deep venous thrombosis, respectively. The probable reasons why these tests are rarely performed are the high risks associated with these invasive procedures and the fairly reliable alternative tests that are available. However, these tests are still repeatedly mentioned in the medical literature as 'gold standards.' Therefore, in the event that a case goes to court because the diagnosis was missed due to one of these alternative tests, the plaintiff attorney will ask why the 'gold standard' was not ordered. The real and substantial risk of the procedure will be irrelevant to the jurors because the diagnosis was missed.

In conclusion, 'gold standard' tests have the greatest sensitivity and/or accuracy. However, they are not always practical in clinical medicine because they may have significant risks, expense, or require great skill to perform. Furthermore, clinicians should not use the results from these tests by themselves and should combine them with their clinical judgment.

Avoid treating children in the same manner as adults

Some physicians believe in the saying, 'kids are just little people.' They believe that they can treat children in the same manner they treat adults. For most situations, this belief will still lead to appropriate treatment. There are instances, however, where failure to appreciate the difference in the child's physiology will lead to an adverse outcome. We also discuss this topic further in the section on airway control in Chapter 10.

Case 4.12 Children are not small adults

Edwards presents a case, in *The M & M Files*, of a 10-year-old boy who was an unrestrained back seat passenger in a motor vehicle accident.[16] He was confused, occasionally drowsy, and agitated and had a laceration on his scalp. The ED physician paralyzed and intubated the patient so that he would be still for the head CT. Intravenous succinylcholine was given without pretreatment with atropine. Before the scan was done, the patient became agitated on two more occasions and was given intravenous succinylcholine on each occasion.

When the patient returned to the ED, his heart rate was less than 30 beats/minute and his blood pressure was unobtainable. He was unable to be resuscitated and the cause of death was believed to be from the medication. His head CT was negative. The physician made an error in not premedicating the child with atropine. Although not routinely performed in adults, atropine is generally recommended in children, especially when multiple doses of succinylcholine are given. This is to prevent the bradycardia that is sometimes induced by succinylcholine. This fatal error was made because of the failure to appreciate the difference in pediatric physiology.

Timothy Kirn of the *Sacramento Bureau* wrote a recent article in *Family Practice News* containing suggestions to avoid malpractice suits in pediatric practice.[17] The article was based on a lecture given by Dr Ramon W Johnson at a pediatric conference. Dr Johnson talked about the '10 commandments' for the reduction of errors in the office pediatric patient. He also discussed some 'red flag situations' to keep in mind.

The '10 commandments' are as follows.

1 Follow stated protocols. This helps avoids gray zones. If you do not follow stated protocols, document why.
2 Use kilograms for weights. This avoids drug errors since most medications are dosed by mg/kg.

3 Have a Broselow tape available. This tape helps the physician save time from computing the drug dosage for a child.
4 Young children should always have their temperature taken rectally. Other routes are just not accurate in this population and fevers in this population cannot be missed.
5 Young children should always have their urine sample obtained by a catheter. Most nurses do not like placing catheters and most parents are afraid to have them placed in their children. They may claim that their doctor does not do it and it is mean to children. As physicians, we must clear up this conception by being consistent and standard. Specimens other than catheter collection or suprapubic aspiration are often contaminated and give false positives.
6 Dr Johnson reiterates what we also endorse. Obtain a pulse oximetry as part of the vital signs.
7 Be careful with decimal points. Many pediatric drug dosages have low numbers and contain decimal points.
8 Maintain the right size equipment. Most adult equipments are too large to be used for children. Furthermore, there is a vast range of sizes among the pediatric age group.
9 'Keep only one concentration of the important medication on hand.'[17]
10 Undress the patient and place them in a gown. A limited physical examination should be performed on all pediatric patients regardless of complaint because of the decreased ability to obtain an accurate history.

Dr Johnson also describes eight 'red flag' situations in the pediatric patient.

1 Be careful with patients who have had a prior visit for the same complaint.
2 Take parents seriously when they say that there has been a behavior change in their child.
3 An inconsolable child who continues to cry in the arms of her parent is ill until proven otherwise.
4 Histories may be confusing and conflicting when a child has multiple caregivers.
5 Children with fever should always be treated with thoroughness and their immunization status must be obtained.
6 Fevers persisting despite antibiotics are even more concerning, particularly for partially treated meningitis due to the poor central nervous system penetration of many antibiotics.
7 Abdominal pain and fever in a child is appendicitis until proven otherwise. This is certainly one of the most popular cases for plaintiff attorneys.
8 Finally, testicular torsion may present in children as abdominal pain.

References

1 Starr DS (2003) Medicine and the Law: A referral would have kept this doctor out of court. *Cortlandt Forum*. **16**(6): 85.
2 Starr DS (2003) Medicine and the Law: Botched neonatal surgery leads to a staggering verdict. *Cortlandt Forum*. **16**(10): 60–61.
3 Starr DS (2003) Medicine and the Law: Botched neonatal surgery leads to a staggering verdict. *Cortlandt Forum*. **16**(10): 61.

4 Cline DM, Ma OJ, Tintinalli JE, Kelen GD and Stapczynski JS (2001) *Just the Facts in Emergency Medicine*. McGraw-Hill, New York, New York, 160.
5 Stark M (1999) Challenging problems presenting as constipation. *American Journal of Gastroenterology*. **94**: 567–74.
6 Edwards FJ (2002) *The M & M Files: morbidity and mortality rounds in emergency medicine*. Hanley & Belfus, Inc., Philadelphia, Pennsylvania, 132–4.
7 Edwards FJ (2002) *The M & M Files: morbidity and mortality rounds in emergency medicine*. Hanley & Belfus, Inc., Philadelphia, Pennsylvania, 132.
8 Starr DS (2003) Medicine and the Law: The foot blister that led to an amputation. *Cortlandt Forum*. **16**(12): 55–6.
9 Starr DS (2003) Medicine and the Law: The foot blister that led to an amputation. *Cortlandt Forum*. **16**(12): 55.
10 Starr DS (2003) Medicine and the Law: The foot blister that led to an amputation. *Cortlandt Forum*. **16**(12): 56.
11 Starr DS (2003) Medicine and the Law: History repeats itself in an obstetrics case. *Cortlandt Forum*. **17**(1): 67–70.
12 Starr DS (2003) Medicine and the Law: History repeats itself in an obstetrics case. *Cortlandt Forum*. **17**(1): 70.
13 Starr DS (2003) Medicine and the Law: How a $1-million award shrank to $100000. *Cortlandt Forum*. **16**(7): 60.
14 Levine C (2004) I was dead wrong. *Medical Economics*. **18**(3): 59–63.
15 Edwards FJ (2002) *The M & M Files: morbidity and mortality rounds in emergency medicine*. Hanley & Belfus, Inc., Philadelphia, Pennsylvania, 217–19.
16 Edwards FJ (2002) *The M & M Files: morbidity and mortality rounds in emergency medicine*. Hanley & Belfus, Inc., Philadelphia, Pennsylvania, 182–3.
17 Kirn TF (2004) Ten ways to inoculate yourself against malpractice suits. *Family Practice News*. **34**(6): 88.

Chapter 5

Dealing with the 'difficult patient'

- The vague patient
- The impatient patient
- The 'one-stop shopping' patient
- The non-compliant patient
- The hostile patient
- The 'VIP' patient
- The predetermined patient
- The seductive patient
- The mentally handicapped patient (e.g. demented, developmentally delayed)
- The psychiatric patient
- The alcohol-intoxicated patient
- The 'drug seeker' patient, the 'frequent flyer' patient
- The anxious patient

The 'difficult patient' has always been a diagnostic and therapeutic challenge for physicians. However, in the current legal environment, the difficult patient can become a high legal risk patient as well. Diagnostic and therapeutic decisions with these patients are hindered by various factors. Although every physician probably has her unique list of patient attributes that she would consider difficult, we have chosen some with which we believe most would concur.

The vague patient

We previously mentioned that the physician must sometimes be a detective. At other times, the physician must play the role of scientist. Medicine is clearly a science and learning it has taught us to be exact and precise in our spoken and written language. We long for the encounter when the patient can tell us exactly when her pain started, every test that has been ordered for her current problem and its result, her list of medications with all of the doses, her immunization record, etc. While we have encountered a few patients who do indeed come to every visit with their complete medical history printed on paper, most patients will not be able to accurately answer every question that is asked of their health. This is usually not a significant detriment to physicians because we are detectives and can usually discern what we need through alternative questioning or other sources.

We will occasionally face a patient who is not contributory or minimally contributory to her history. This type of patient may answer that her symptoms have been present 'for a while' or that 'it just hurts' when asked to describe the nature of her pain. Some will just state that they are 'sick' or 'don't feel good' and leave further interpretation to the physician. With these patients, you may try to ask questions from different angles, using frequent closed-ended questions, or obtaining the history from alternative sources. If these further attempts yield no additional clue to the patient's problem, you must rely on the physical exam. When the physical exam is noncontributory, consider the 'grope-o-gram.' The 'grope-o-gram' is a set of tests designed to detect general medical abnormalities. The set usually include a complete blood count, a basic metabolic panel, and a urinalysis. It may also include a chest X-ray, an electrocardiogram, a head CT, and drug levels.

After the history, physical exam, and diagnostic tests are completed, the physician should have some direction to the nature of the patient's problem. However, if the diagnosis is still uncertain, consider admission for observation, close follow-up, or referral for consultation or further testing. In addition, consider alternate diagnoses like psychiatric conditions or chronic conditions like HIV or cancer. We have found that electrolyte abnormalities, occult cancers, HIV infection, and thyroid dysfunction are frequent illnesses that produce clinical manifestations that are difficult for patients to explain.

Case 5.1 Symptoms that are difficult to pinpoint

Edwards describes, in *The M & M Files*, the case of a cranky 63-year-old man with a history of chronic obstructive pulmonary disease and hypertension who presented to the emergency department with multiple complaints including shortness of breath and shakiness.[1] The ED physician was annoyed to see the multiple complaints. He engaged in an argument with the patient why he had not seen his primary physician for these problems. The doctor performed his examination and proceeded to order a complete blood count, chest X-ray, and a nebulizer treatment with albuterol and Atrovent. The patient's breathing became slightly better. He was discharged with an antibiotic and instructed to see his primary physician.

The patient returned to the ED the following day with worsening symptoms. A different ED physician ordered a metabolic panel and discovered that the patient was a new-onset type II diabetic with a blood-glucose of 870 mg/dl. The medical pearl is to consider electrolyte imbalance when patients present with vague symptoms involving multiple organ systems. Always consider an organic cause for multiple complaints before attributing them to the patient's personality.

The impatient patient

Most people have busy and tight schedules (physicians and patients). Almost every service requires a waiting time that can sometimes be prolonged depending on the provider's schedule. Although no one enjoys the inconvenience of waiting, most will understand if a reasonable explanation of the delay is given. Some patients, however, have impatience that is extremely difficult to pacify.

These patients may have a great sense of grandiosity and believe that their time is more valuable than that of others. This behavior makes them difficult to treat because they can be hostile, unreasonable, and averse to evaluations that require any significant amount of time.

We feel the best approach for the physician is to apologize for the delay, give patients an explanation for the delay, and then treat in the normal fashion. Whether patients accept or reject the explanation, we are not persistent at appeasing patients if we have been preoccupied with treating other patients in an orderly fashion. Delays are a natural aspect of business. Although some patients will continue to complain and fuss during the history taking and physical, the physician should stay objective and perform the evaluation as usual. Physicians should avoid letting the patient's frustration affect the medical evaluation because it is not professional or medically wise.

The impatient patient may be reluctant to take off her clothes and may also refuse certain tests because of time restraints. The physician should not concede to these objections without explaining to the patient why the recommendations were made. If she still refuses, then document her reasoning as to the recommendations and her subsequent refusal. Remember that the impatient patient should be offered the same evaluation as the patient who is patient and receptive to your care. This is the principle behind professionalism and will decrease medical liability.

At times, the impatient patient will be courteous and friendly. She may try to dissuade the physician from ordering certain tests because of time constraints. Although this patient may seem to be a low medical liability risk patient, this presumption may be false if an important test is not ordered. If she leaves and has an adverse outcome because a test was not done, her reason for leaving becomes secondary to the physician's incomplete evaluation. In addition, although she may not have sounded like the litigious type during the visit, she may change her tune after she has undergone medical suffering. Furthermore, there are plenty of large billboards, commercials, and advertisements of malpractice lawyers encouraging her to come for a consultation. (We have also read stories about malpractice lawyers planting 'spies' in hospitals as orderly, techs, and other employees to search for business).

A good example is the low-risk patient who presents with chest pain. The low-risk patient complains of chest pain symptoms that are atypical with acute coronary syndrome. She may have one or even two risk factors. Her initial EKG and cardiac enzymes are normal. However, in patients who present within six to eight hours of the onset of the pain, or are still having pain, we generally like to perform serial EKGs and cardiac enzymes at least three hours apart. This may help us detect an evolving acute coronary syndrome. These patients will sometimes request to go home when their initial tests are normal. However, early discharges of these patients also represent a significant percentage of the missed myocardial infarctions that have plagued emergency physicians. Tolerability for missed myocardial infarctions is extremely low among the public, attorneys, courts, and even the medical profession because of the grave consequences. Therefore, do your patient and yourself the favor of completing the necessary evaluations before you let them go home. Physicians should encourage their patients to be patient and complete the necessary tests.

The 'one-stop shopping' patient

Everyone wants to economize their time. Hence, it is not unusual for a patient to present multiple problems to her physician on a single visit. This happens frequently in primary care practices that are relatively busy and where it is difficult for patients to get timely appointments. It also occurs in urgent care patients and in emergency patients who seldom visit doctors until they have accumulated multiple problems.

Unfortunately, these patients become problematic due to the time constraints caused by managed care and emergency department overcrowding. These patients may come with a shopping list of complaints or answer the question of 'what has been bothering you?' with the response, 'everything.' Most physicians will agree that they were taught as medical students that most visits (excluding annual physicals) should last less than 15 minutes. This length of time is usually sufficient for an experienced physician to address all of the patient's problems. The dilemma arises when the current legal environment is taken into consideration. Each complaint requires a set of questions on the history, examinations on the physicals, and specific tests in order to complete a well-documented chart. For example, a patient may come with an ingrown toenail but states, 'I also have a headache.' This last statement mandates questioning for secondary causes of headaches (e.g. subarachnoid hemorrhage) and a neurologic examination. Hence, it can become frustrating to treat patients with multiple complaints.

The best advice with these types of patients is that if time allows, address each separate problem as if it is a presenting complaint. However, most physicians do not have the time to evaluate more than a couple of problems on each visit. If the physician is confident that a particular problem does not represent an emergency (e.g. a visit for medication refills or lab work), then arranging a follow-up appointment to address the problem is appropriate. The art is to not make the patient feel that she is ignored. However, if there is any doubt, then it is best to address the problem. This prevents the physician from having to respond to the famous quote 'my doctor did not listen to me' later in the courtroom.

The non-compliant patient

We all have these types of patients in our practices and our own stories of how difficult they can be. They do not adhere to our recommendations. They are also hard to follow clinically because they do not keep track of their medications and comply with scheduled tests. Consequently, their non-compliance occasionally results in adverse consequences and high medical liability for the treating physician. Although every practice consists of non-compliant patients, there is increased prevalence in the emergency department, where lack of regular care, lack of physician trust, and lack of finances are more frequent contributing factors.

Do not develop a safeguard in believing that you are not responsible for your patient's non-compliance. The public, attorneys, judges, and jurors expect physicians (as they probably should) to be parental figures to their patients. This means that physicians should use every reasonable measure to help patients take care of their own health. Examples include: finding affordable medicines (or giving samples), sending out reminders for appointments and tests, scheduling more frequent visits, etc. In short, make the effort to correct any factors contributing to the non-compliance and document these efforts in the chart. If the patient is still resistant and the message is not getting through, then we recommend that you consider terminating the relationship. Warn the patient that you feel that you may not be the right doctor for the patient. This may seem extreme to some physicians and not in conformity with the 'traditional doctors' of the past. However, we feel that it is necessary because of the current legal environment. Our beloved forefathers in medicine did not lived in the same legal environment in which we live today. Remember, our emergency department colleagues do not have the alternative of discharging patients from their practice and can tell great stories of how problematic these patients can become.

Case 5.2 Will this patient just listen?

One particular patient who we treat regularly in the emergency department gives a classic example of how non-compliance affects the patient evaluation. A 60-year-old gentleman sees us at least once every two weeks for the past two years for multiple pain complaints for which he demands narcotics. Interestingly, his wife does the exact same thing. The majority of this gentleman's pain visits are for low back pain. Unfortunately, he is a heavy smoker (non-compliant with repeated urges to quit) with a history of untreated hypertension (non-compliant with medications). On his first visit for low back pain, we ordered a CT scan of his abdomen, which confirmed our suspicion for an abdominal aortic aneurysm of 5.4 cm in diameter. The dilemma now arises. Every two weeks when he returns for low back pain and states that the pain is worsening, does the current visit warrant a repeat CT scan for dissection or rupture? It does not help that he refuses to see a vascular surgeon for the problem or stop smoking as advised. A lot of money is being spent on a non-compliant patient. We do order repeat CT scans on every visit that he states the pain is worse. Whether he is 'crying wolf' to get more narcotics or he actually does have an acute emergency is difficult to determine on clinical examination. He may present one day with a ruptured or leaking aneurysm and die because of his non-compliance. We hope that the emergency physician on duty that day does not treat him like another drug seeker because we do not feel that the jury will accept the patient's non-compliance as an excuse for missing a ruptured aneurysm.

The hostile patient

Hostile patients are difficult to treat. They also represent a safety concern for the treating physician and other staff members. The most important concept to remember is not to become engaged in the patient's hostility. Arguing or fighting with the patient will demonstrate a lack of control to the other patients and to the staff. In contrast, the maintenance of a calm demeanor will show the patient that his or her hostility has not affected your medical judgment. Remain objective because these patients will be of equal or even greater risk of initiating legal action for any adverse outcome.

As the physician, you should assure the safety of yourself and your staff. Always make sure that there is adequate manpower in case the patient becomes violent. Do not leave a female nurse in a room alone with a hostile patient. Alert anyone that may interact with the patient of the potential for hostility. Remember, if you do not take these measures and one of your staff gets injured, you may be involved in a non-malpractice related lawsuit.

Some of the safety measures implemented in the emergency department to ensure staff safety are as follows.

1 Avoid bringing anything into the patient room that may be used as a weapon (e.g. knife, fork, extra needles, etc.).
2 Fully undress the patient so that there are no hidden weapons.
3 Alert security for the potential of hostility and violence.
4 Order sedation if patient is combative before requesting testing.
5 Minimize the interaction of hostile patients with other patients and families (e.g. shorten the time in the waiting room).

The 'VIP' patient

Although we will admit that there are quite a few individuals in our own profession who believe that they are 'God's gift' to medicine, we occasionally come across a patient who is equally (or even more) arrogant. These patients have a sense of grandiosity and expect the VIP ('very important person') treatment. They may demand a particular test or treatment to make them 'get better quicker' or say that 'I can't afford to be sick.' They may expect to be given antibiotics for viral illnesses, demand immediate tests for non-emergent conditions (e.g. ultrasound for cholelithiasis), or insist on a specialist to be called immediately (e.g. plastic surgeon for a routine hand laceration).

Although each physician has her own way of handling these patients based on her personality, our rule of thumb is to try to pacify them as much as possible as long as their request is reasonable. That is to say we would not give them antibiotics if we were absolutely confident that the infection was viral. If there is any concern of a bacterial infection, however, the threshold for dispensing antibiotics is lower. In the case of gallbladder pain, an emergent ultrasound is ordered if there is any suspicion of acute cholecystitis, whereas if it is clearly a case of simple biliary colic, we try to arrange a non-emergent ultrasound for the patient as soon as possible. As far as requests for calling specialists, we usually comply with these because a phone call is inexpensive and does no harm. There is no guarantee given to the patient that a phone call will mean that the specialist will come treat the patient if it is a problem that she feels the treating physician can competently manage. However, we have seen time and time again, physicians have been reprimanded by administration, health agencies, and lawyers for not making a 'simple phone call.' The underlying principle with all patients, these in particular, is that they are still our customers and we should try to give service to their satisfaction that is within medical reason.

<hr>

Case 5.3 Who are we treating here?

Our best case of the VIP patient is actually not of the patient but that of her husband. A middle-aged female with a history of chronic gastrointestinal blood loss presented to the emergency department requesting a blood transfusion. She had been fully worked up by her own gastroenterologist and refused another evaluation. When her hemoglobin was confirmed to be low, we discussed the case with our gastroenterologist on call. He recommended that we transfuse her with two units of packed red blood cells and discharge her. The husband became outraged at this proposition and wanted her admitted to the hospital for the transfusion. He stated that he 'was a very important man and had a schedule that was much busier' than ours. He did not want his wife admitted because he was concerned for her medical condition. Rather, he wanted her admitted so he could go home and not miss work the following morning. Although we were offended by this man's arrogance, we handled it professionally and called the gastroenterologist who decided to admit her.

<hr>

The predetermined patient

Some patients will come to see you only because they need your license to obtain what they feel they need. These patients are usually sure what their diagnosis is and they want certain medicines to treat it or tests to confirm it. Many claim to have read a lot of literature or researched extensively on the Internet on a certain problem or discussed it with a 'doctor' family member or friend. They are determined to adhere to their preconceived notions about their illness and can sometimes be resistant to your opinions.

The two most common examples in our practices are the patient with a viral illness who is adamant about receiving an antibiotic to 'nip it in the bud', and the headache patient who insists that they need a head CT. These patients are best handled on a case-by-case basis. Your evaluation must proceed objectively in your usual fashion. Then you must compare and analyze what you feel is best for the patient with what the patient feels is best for them. Then add the intangible factor of whether the particular patient involved will accept your opinion and the likelihood of their following your instructions.

If the patient requests tests that are not harmful or costly, it may be best to order the tests. This gesture frequently leads to greater patient satisfaction. For tests that involve some risks (e.g. intravenous contrast, radiation) or are fairly expensive (e.g. CT scan, MRI) that you do not feel that the patient needs, make sure that you explain these cons to the patient to try to dissuade the patient. If unsuccessful, it becomes your discretion whether to order these tests. Just keep in mind that medicine is extremely bureaucratic today and sometimes it is not whether you perform good medicine or not but whether you please the patient.

Case 5.4 Complaints will come even when you do everything right

We saw a 50-year-old woman in the emergency department. She presented with 12 hours of diffuse abdominal pain and multiple bouts of nausea and vomiting. She also had three episodes of syncope. Her past medical history was significant for previous surgery for a tubo-ovarian abscess. She stated repeatedly that she was suffering from food poisoning.

On physical examination, she was hypotensive with a blood pressure of 90/46 mm Hg. Her abdominal examination revealed diffuse tenderness and mild guarding. Pelvic and rectal examinations were performed and were unremarkable. Her white blood cell count was elevated at 12 000 cells/microliter with a left shift of 12% bands.

Our differential diagnoses included gastroenteritis, food poisoning, appendicitis, pancreatitis, tubo-ovarian abscess, diverticulitis, cholecystitis, and ruptured abdominal aortic aneurysm. In addition to the complete blood count, we ordered serum chemistries, liver functions, amylase, lipase, and a CT scan of the abdomen and pelvis. With the exception of the complete blood count, the other test results were normal. She was treated successfully for acute gastroenteritis.

Two years later, she filed a complaint to the State Board of Health against us. She felt that the pelvic and rectal exams were unnecessary. We replied that it was explained to her that a pelvic exam was performed for two reasons. It should be done in any female with lower abdominal pain. It should also be checked for a patient with a prior history of tubo-ovarian abscess. As for the rectal exam, she was told the four reasons why it was needed. She had suspected gastroenteritis and we needed to check the stool for blood. Likewise, we needed to check her stool for blood because of the abdominal pain. She had an episode of syncope and the evaluation should include a search for occult blood loss. Finally, she was hypotensive and this also requires a search for blood loss.

The second part of her complaint was that excessive tests were ordered. She felt that the only tests that were necessary were a complete blood count and stool cultures. We pointed out the numerous red flags that this patient had and provided medical literature to support every test and exam that we performed. We also provided literature stating the recommended criteria for the appropriateness of stool cultures. This patient did not meet any of these criteria. However, since stool cultures are harmless and not costly, we would have probably ordered them if she had made the request.

This case reminded us of how difficult the predetermined patient can be. Although the physician may follow the standard of care, the treatment may not be consistent with the patient's predetermined conceptions. The physician should try to perform an evaluation that is to the patient's satisfaction. More importantly, the physician should never alter the standard of care. These concepts not only help decrease the possibility of adverse outcomes, they will help the physician respond to complaints in a professional and evidence-based fashion.

The same can be said concerning the prescription of requested medications. From our experience, however, unnecessary medications have a greater probability of causing harm (e.g. allergic reactions, antibiotics masking occult infections) than unnecessary diagnostic tests and mandate greater caution in their dispensing. The physician should assess the certainty of each patient's diagnosis. If there is any doubt about the patient's diagnosis, it may be better to honor the patient's request. For example, it may be better to prescribe antibiotics to the patient with an unclear source of fever. In this situation, the patient is more likely to take legal action if they become worse without the antibiotics. In addition, they will probably be more willing to accept an adverse drug reaction.

The seductive patient

This is a problem that is present in any occupation with significant people interaction. However, it is especially prevalent in medicine where patients come to the physician seeking care and empathy. Some may be subtle with their intentions, such as repeated visits, while others are overt and may stalk the physician. A friend of ours in the emergency department had one female that would persistently call almost every night to find out if he was working.

While these patients usually do not mean any physical harm, their behavior could affect your medical evaluation. Engaging in a personal relationship with the patient will make it difficult for the physician to evaluate the patient objectively. Furthermore, a seductive patient may not give an accurate history and omit details that they feel may upset their physician. They may also create problems to obtain more attention and not accept referrals to another physician.

Physicians should treat these patients objectively. Avoid anything that will give the patient the impression that she is being treated differently. Do not concede to her requests for unnecessary appointments. If she comes to the emergency department, ask another physician to treat her. When examining these patients, bring a chaperone. Finally, have nurses screen phone calls and messages from these patients to prevent non-medical conversations.

The mentally handicapped patient (e.g. demented, developmentally delayed)

These patients are difficult to obtain a history from or perform a physical examination on. Their abilities to give helpful accounts of their illnesses are often limited or non-existent. However, do not automatically assume that they cannot give a history and assess their alertness and orientation. It may be imperative to utilize ancillary personnel (e.g. family, care-givers, paramedics, etc.) to get a good account of the patient's illness. Additional information may be obtained by searching the charts for other contacts of the patient.

Physical examination may also be limited due to the patient's impaired ability to follow instructions. Useful information may be elicited from other members of the medical staff who are involved in the patient's care. For example, the patient may not move her extremities for you but may move them when the nurse attempts to place an intravenous line. Therefore, examinations by committee will yield more physical findings than an examination by a single physician. Certain parts of the physical exam are more difficult to perform in these patients. The patient may not relax her legs for a pelvic examination. In these cases, alternative methods may be required (e.g. sedation before a pelvic exam). The important concept to remember is that evaluation of these patients may take extra effort and should not rest on the complacency of only doing the things that are convenient.

The psychiatric patient

These patients are difficult to manage for several reasons. Their complaints may be absurd, involve multiple organ systems, and have no medical basis. In this aspect, they can be as difficult to treat as the 'one-stop shopping patient' discussed above. Their histories can ramble on and on in a tangential fashion without any orderly sequence. They may have past medical problems that are not well taken care of or well described. In addition, they may be treated with multiple psychiatric medications and have undergone multiple surgeries. Finally, their physical exam may reveal findings that are self-induced and conversion reactions.

They may seek or demand care that is detrimental to them. We are all familiar with the Munchausen's syndrome patient who thrives on having extensive tests and procedures performed on her. With these patients, giving them what they want or request may not only cause them further physical injury but also mentally handicap them into believing that they do have organic causes for their symptoms.

Case 5.5 Sometimes you have to say no

We saw a 23-year-old healthy male with no medical history who presented with the chief complaint: 'wants cardiac surgery tonight.' He had absolutely nothing wrong with his heart but had a psychiatric history. He was disappointed when we decided to treat him medically and not surgically.

Dealing with the new onset psychiatric patient is especially challenging. A thorough medical evaluation is essential to rule out organic causes. This may include a CT scan of the head, a drug screen, serum electrolytes, and evaluation for sources of infection (e.g. chest X-ray, urinalysis, cerebrospinal fluid). A lumbar puncture to obtain cerebrospinal fluid is frequently indicated. Informing the patient or her family of a psychiatric condition is no easy task. Making a disposition on these patients may also be difficult. Psychiatric facilities are limited and many patients are unwilling to be treated. Finally, it is not always easy to determine if a patient needs involuntary hospitalization.

The suicidal patient is a special subset of the psychiatric patients because of the additional legal implications. Physicians sometimes find themselves in a 'Catch-22' situation. We are required, by law, to involuntarily hospitalize patients whom we feel may present danger to themselves or to others. We are all familiar with the case of the suicidal patient (or the potentially suicidal patient) who was not hospitalized. This patient subsequently committed suicide a few days later and the family sued for an exorbitant amount. For this reason, our advice is to complete a Baker Act (involuntary hospitalization) for anyone that you have any doubts about. Indeed, the law protects physicians from any repercussions from involuntarily hospitalizing a patient if the physician has good documentation to show her concern for the patient's safety. However, patients (and sometimes their families) are rarely happy with involuntary hospitalization. Therefore, they will occasionally try to create legal problems for the physician.

Case 5.6 Not giving in to threats

We had a case involving a middle-aged female with a history of cancer and depression. She had multiple suicide attempts in the past. She presented to our emergency department one afternoon after a couple of empty pill bottles (which were not hers) were found in her bathroom. She admitted that this was a suicide attempt to the paramedics, the triage nurse, and to us. Her significant other came shortly afterwards and wanted to take her home with her. She stated that she had called the patient's primary physician and he told her that the patient could go home because she had done this in the past. We, along with the rest of the emergency department staff, strongly felt that this patient was a danger to herself. Because she refused psychiatric evaluation on the encouragement of her partner, we were forced to complete a Baker Act form. Her partner immediately became outraged and threatened legal action against us. This did not alter our management plans because our priority was to protect the patient (and our medical license).

Three months later, we received a letter from our state health agency stating that we were under investigation for non-professional medical conduct. This investigation was based on a complaint from the patient's outraged significant other. Although we understand that state health agencies are obligated to investigate every patient complaint, this one had no legal or medical foundation. We also felt that part of the problem was that the patient's primary physician acted inappropriately in telling the patient's partner that she could go home when he did not evaluate her during the current situation. After writing a long letter to explain our position and also having other witnesses from the emergency department corroborate our findings during that visit, the state health agency terminate the investigation.

The alcohol-intoxicated patient

These patients are difficult to manage because they can manifest a potpourri of undesirable personality traits including anger, combativeness, confusion, and impatience. Much of what has been previously discussed in the preceding paragraph could also pertain to the patient who is intoxicated with alcohol.

They often give an inaccurate history of their alcohol use and are sometimes in denial. We had one patient whom we asked, 'Do you drink heavily?' He responded, 'What do you consider heavy?' He then proceeded to tell us that he drank 'every day and every night' and drank 'this morning to prevent my shakes.' The alcoholic patient may object to treatment in the same manner that the above patients do. However, the physician must use careful judgment in deciding whether the alcoholic patient is capable of making her own decisions. If in doubt, err on the side of an incompetent patient and commit her to involuntary treatment (i.e. Marchment Act). You still may be reviewed for this action (by State Health Agencies or Hospital Committees) but you are much less likely to have a malpractice suit against you.

In the event that the intoxicated patient is a chronic alcoholic (which is frequently the case), she is more inclined to have serious underlying medical conditions or be more prone to develop certain medical conditions. Alcoholics are usually malnourished which makes their wound healing more difficult. They also tend to take poor care of their health and seldom have a private physician. These factors increase their likelihood of having undetected medical illnesses and immunization and nutritional deficiencies. Liver disease, seizures, coagulopathy, pancreatic disease, and cancers are all more commonly found in alcoholics. Because of their tendency to fall, alcoholics are also prone to develop subdural hematomas. The combination of alcohol-induced gastric irritation and coagulopathy makes alcoholics susceptible to peptic ulcer disease, gastritis, gastrointestinal bleeding, and Mallory–Weiss tears.

The alcoholic patient also presents numerous social dilemmas. They frequently live alone or are homeless, thus, making discharge dispositions difficult. Accompanying psychiatric conditions are not uncommon and may need to be addressed concurrently (e.g. they may have been trying to 'drink themselves to death'). They may present health risks to others or to themselves upon discharge (may drive while still intoxicated or may walk in front of a car). Some may even leave before they are discharged as in the case below. Finally, they may be at high risk for alcohol withdrawal upon discharge.

It is obvious that suicidal, homicidal, or delusional patients need to be guarded from leaving because of the potential risks to themselves and to others. However, guarding an intoxicated patient from leaving the ED is not routinely done. This is because most intoxicated patients do not have intentions of hurting themselves or hurting others. Furthermore, most intoxicated patients know that they will get better with intravenous fluids and do not wish to leave the ED. Once the patient does leave, however, they may still come into harm's way because of their impaired mentation.

Case 5.7 Watch them like a hawk

Edwards presents another case from *The M & M Files* of an intoxicated patient who endangered himself.[2] An intoxicated 35-year-old man came to the ED requesting treatment and placement into a detoxification center. He was from out of town and did not have anywhere else to go. The ED physician examined him and found no signs of alcohol withdrawal. After

---

continued

a blood alcohol level came back at 150 mg/dl, the physician asked the social worker to help the patient with placement.

As he was waiting for placement, the patient was moved to a quiet room. Later, another intoxicated patient came in for a scalp laceration. After his laceration was repaired, he was also moved into the quiet room to wait until his friend could pick him up. When placement into a detoxification center was arranged for the first patient 30 minutes later, the physician went to the quiet room to find that it was empty.

An ambulance brought the first patient back several hours later. The patient was following the new friend that he had met in the quiet room to a bar when a vehicle hit him as he was running across the interstate. He had a severe head injury and was pronounced dead on arrival. His family filed a lawsuit against the physician and the hospital for failing to protect him. The initial verdict was for the patient's family but was later overturned.

This case is not too uncommon and lawsuits of this nature typically occur against hospitals and restaurants. Both institutions are frequently charged with allowing an impaired client to walk into the dangers of the street. The physician and the hospital had to go through great expense and stress to fight the above claim. We do not feel that they were negligent in protecting the patient's safety. A blood alcohol level of 150 mg/dl is not one for which we keep patients in the ED (typically greater than 300 mg/dl). Otherwise, the crowded ED dilemma in the United States would be even worse than it currently is. The medical staff did its best to arrange appropriate disposition for the patient. In retrospect, placing two intoxicated patients together was probably not a good idea, but this would have been difficult to predict. The patient could also have been kept in the immediate view of the ED staff. In our opinion, if the patient was competent enough to request alcohol detoxification, then he was competent enough to choose to leave the ED.

Patients with heavy alcohol use will often present to the emergency department after trauma (e.g. motor vehicle accidents, falls with head injuries). This is an especially high-risk medical situation because they are unable to give accurate histories of their injuries. Their intoxication can also mask clinical exam findings.

Case 5.8 Raising the height of suspicion

There was a case of an intoxicated restrained driver in a motor vehicle accident who had no complaints of abdominal pain and had no apparent tenderness or masses on abdominal examination. He was slightly hypotensive, which was believed to be from the alcohol. He was observed for several hours in the emergency department as his blood pressure improved with fluids and then released only to become hypotensive from a retroperitoneal hemorrhage 30 minutes after discharge. In fact, there are some physicians who recommend an abdominal CT scan in hypotensive trauma patients who are intoxicated. In these situations, the reliability of the abdominal exam is limited.

Alcohol intoxication should never be assumed to be the etiology of serious physical findings until other causes have been excluded.

Case 5.9 Alcohol intoxication is a diagnosis of exclusion

In *Preventing Malpractice Lawsuits in Pediatric Emergency Medicine* by Selbst and Korin, a man's unconsciousness was mistakenly attributed to alcohol.[3] An intoxicated man with a history of diabetes was taken to an emergency department following a motor vehicle accident. He received a blood alcohol level but no other diagnostic tests. When he awoke and was combative, he was moved into an observation room to let the alcohol subside.

A few hours later, he went into cardiac arrest and died. The patient had not been taken off the spinal immobilization board and was still fully dressed. On autopsy, it was discovered that his arrest originated from blunt chest trauma with accompanying lacerations to his lung and his aorta. A lawsuit was filed against the ED staff and resulted in a $2 million settlement. The physician in this case made a huge assumption that alcohol was the cause of this patient's lethargy, and later, combativeness. This assumption should never be made in the presence of other factors such as diabetes and with major trauma.

The 'drug seeker' patient, the 'frequent flyer' patient

Almost all physicians have these types of patients in their practice. This is because these patients have no typical demographic characteristic. They may be rich or poor, young or old, male or female, and of any nationality. We group the two together because they are often one in the same; that is to say, they require frequent visits to obtain more pain medicines. They commonly present to the emergency department or the urgent care center. At these centers, patients feel more comfortable because their medication use and/or visit history are usually unknown to the treating physician. Even on the occasion when the physician is familiar with the patient, there is still less than optimal information on the patient.

Childress offers tips on how to identify drug-seeking patients in an article from *Physicians Practice*.[4]

1 Vague symptoms of pain.
2 Conditions which are difficult to prove or disprove – low back pain, neck pain, migraine, renal colic, toothache.
3 Pain that doesn't make sense; symptoms that don't add up.
4 Requests for medication by name and dose.
5 Medical knowledge beyond the realm of what you see in the average patient.
6 Allergies to nearly everything – except the drug of choice.
7 Patient calls ahead to see who is on duty at the clinic, ED, or urgent care center.
8 'Bad-mouthing' previous physicians.
9 Hesitant to follow through with a work-up to get to bottom of a problem.

10 Losing prescriptions or medications.
11 Alert from a pharmacy or insurance that a patient is getting meds from several sources.

These patients are difficult to treat due to multiple reasons. Their medical file may be scattered among many different offices and emergency departments (making it difficult to track their prescriptions). They usually present with pain complaints such as headaches, dental pain, and back pain, which are all difficult to gauge objectively. It is not uncommon for these patients to be 'allergic' to multiple medicines (i.e. all non-narcotic pain medicines) and be demanding of specific medicines. Finally, they may give false information because some of them have criminal records or do not want to be traced. We participated in a study concerning pain management in dental pain. We called patients who we treated for dental pain to see how their pain was two days from the initial visit. One of the conclusions that we made from this study was that almost half of the patients in the study gave false demographic information and were lost to follow-up. The sample size of the study, however, was extremely small.

There are many potential pitfalls that physicians should be cognizant of when treating these patients. Having been labeled as a 'drug seeker' or 'frequent flyer', these patients automatically receive a negative image from the medical staff. Staff members will often warn the physician that 'patient is here again', and 'for the same old reason.' These comments should not lower the physician's guard for emergent conditions. Examine the patient with as much objectivity as possible and avoid a cursory examination, which is often given for patients who come frequently. Avoid the temptation to bypass the routine steps that you would normally follow because of suggestions from your staff that the 'patient has the same old problem.' Remember, most physicians have the clinical skills and knowledge to avoid making medical mistakes. However, details may be overlooked when steps are skipped.

The anxious patient

Most patients have some degree of anxiety during the medical visit. This is almost a normal reaction to the role of being 'sick.' However, the patient with extreme anxiety may become problematic in many different ways. The following discussion pertains to anxious patients without an underlying psychiatric disorder.

The anxious patient may complain of many different symptoms involving various organ systems. They may also present their symptoms without any chronological order or present them in a dramatic fashion. Open-ended questions generally are not effective because of their nebulous responses. The histories they give may frustrate and confuse the physician, especially one that is under a time limitation.

Obtaining a good history from these patients is still important. It may be beneficial to use closed-ended questions and maintain the direction of the interview. Patient reassurance, time out, sedative medications, or having another individual obtain the history are alternatives to try in refractory cases. Patients are sometimes more at ease in talking with a nurse or a medical assistant.

Case 5.10 Having patience with patients

Edwards presents a case, in *The M & M Files*, where the patient's anxiety was used as an excuse for obtaining a poor history.[5] Two days after falling while lifting boxes, a 56-year-old obese woman came to the emergency department for treatment. The patient had a history of nonspecific back pain and was now complaining of diffuse spinal pain from the neck to the tailbone.

The physician stated on the chart that he had difficulty examining the patient because of her anxiety and her diffuse symptoms. There were very few details in the chart on the mechanism of her injury. Her physical exam did not reveal any sensory or motor deficits and her lumbar spine seemed to have the most tenderness. After interpreting her lumbosacral X-rays as negative, the physician discharged her with medications for pain and muscle spasms.

The patient had a repeat visit to the ED two weeks later. She now had increased pain in her back and neck and it was associated with weakness in her arms and legs. Her right arm was too weak for her to use the crutches that her primary physician had prescribed. She also complained of several episodes of urinary incontinence and inability to feel the needle of her insulin injections. A second ED physician examined her and noted that she was a 'tough historian' who was anxious and weepy.[6] The physician also commented that the patient was uncooperative with the physical examination and attributed these new symptoms to the patient's anxiety and repeated the lumbosacral X-rays with the same results. The patient was then medicated and discharged with instructions to follow up with her physician. She had to be carried to her car.

Several days later, she went to another facility and received a MRI of her spine. This revealed that she had a large cervical disk herniation. She was left with disabling neurological deficits after surgery and physical therapy. A lawsuit was filed against the ED physicians at the first facility. The history recorded at this facility stated that the patient fell off a step-ladder, struck the back of her head on some boxes and hyperflexed her neck.

The two ED physicians who treated this patient allowed the patient's anxiety to hinder their evaluations. Adequate histories and examinations were not performed because she was considered a 'difficult patient.' The evaluations might have been more fruitful if the physicians had considered sedating the patient or allowed her the necessary time for her anxiety to improve.

References

1   Edwards FJ (2002) *The M & M Files: morbidity and mortality rounds in emergency medicine.* Hanley & Belfus Inc., Philadelphia, Pennsylvania, 30–32.

2   Edwards FJ (2002) *The M & M Files: morbidity and mortality rounds in emergency medicine.* Hanley & Belfus Inc., Philadelphia, Pennsylvania, 203–4.

3   Selbst SM and Korin JB (1999) *Preventing Malpractice Lawsuits in Pediatric Emergency Medicine.* American College of Emergency Physicians, Dallas, Texas, 119–20.

4   Childress K (2004) Drug-seeking patients: how to spot them, treat them, and protect your practice. *Physicians Practice.* **14**(6): 50.*

5   Edwards FJ (2002) *The M & M Files: morbidity and mortality rounds in emergency medicine.* Hanley & Belfus Inc., Philadelphia, Pennsylvania, 170–172.

6   Edwards FJ (2002) *The M & M Files: morbidity and mortality rounds in emergency medicine.* Hanley & Belfus Inc., Philadelphia, Pennsylvania, 170.

Chapter 6

Clinical tips to decrease liability in your practice: part 1

- Practice good medicine
- Assure good turnover of patients at shift change
- Help your nurses prevent medication errors
- Help yourself prevent medication errors
- Be well read and trained
- Know your medical terms
- Do not give the impression that you work for the pharmaceutical companies
- Develop 'standards of practice'
- Physicians should address non-emergent but potentially serious problems
- Be careful about prescribing medicines to a patient without examining them
- Serve as a good citizen
- Give returning patients a step-up in evaluation
- Be proud and supportive of your profession
- Assume your chart documentation will be read by others
- Complete your medical notes and documents in a timely fashion
- Develop peer review of charts in your practice
- Be your worst critic
- Utilize telephone follow-ups with your patients
- Respect other physicians
- Make effective use of consultants
- Be well read on medical-legal cases and issues
- Know about your medications
- Be careful when selecting partners for your practice
- Be careful when selecting employees for your practice
- Follow treatment guidelines and protocols

Practice good medicine

It goes without saying that practicing good medicine is probably your best chance to avoid a lawsuit. What 'good medicine' entails can be interpreted in many ways. We feel that 'good medicine' is giving medical care that is within or beyond the 'standard of care' for each particular medical problem. That is, doing the same thing as the majority of your equally trained peers would do in the same situation.

Good medicine includes a caring and courteous bedside manner and an excellent rapport with patients. We have all been told that patients are less likely to initiate a suit against you if they like you. The corollary to this is that patients are also more likely to accept an adverse outcome or mistake if you showed them you cared in their health treatment. Before you discharge a patient, talk to them concerning your final assessment and answer any questions that they may have. It is easy to evaluate a patient, give a medication order, and then discharge a patient. However, our experience is that patients are most satisfied when they are given a closing conversation with their treating physician. Do not discharge a patient that is unsure of their diagnosis or has a blank stare on his or her face because he or she is not likely to follow your directions or be happy with your care.

Horn *et al.* cited a study, in *Law For Physicians: an overview of medical legal issues*, that examined behaviors in patient claims and concluded that 'problems with communication between physicians and patients were often crucial factors in precipitating individuals to file suit.'[1] Patients cited the following as common reasons for putting forth a claim. Their physician either did not want to talk or listen to them. Their physician misled them. Finally, their physician used terminology that they could not understand.

Another study in 1997 from the *Journal of the American Medical Association* demonstrated that physicians without previous claims 'used more statements of orientation (educating patients about what to expect and the flow of a visit), laughed and used humor more,…tended to use more facilitation (soliciting patients' opinions, checking understanding, and encouraging patients to talk) [, and…] spent longer in routine visits.'[2]

Finally, good medicine means that you educate your patients. Remember, the definition of 'doctor' in the dictionary includes 'teacher.'[3] Although it is difficult to overcome the time constraints of physicians' practices today to spend as much time educating patients as we would like, there are several methods to inform your patients without placing more burden on your schedule. These include using preprinted information sheets on particular diseases, referring your patients to internet reference sites, or having a staff member answer the patient's questions in further detail. In addition, you can use referrals to ancillary specialists such as nutritionists, physical therapists, etc.

You must realize, however, that practicing good medicine does not ensure that you will not be named in a malpractice suit. As Horn *et al.* write, in *Law For Physicians: an overview of medical legal issues*, there are multiple other factors that could contribute to a lawsuit that are not related to a physician's clinical competence. 'First, everyone makes mistakes. None of us is on top of the game 100 percent of the time.'[4] Mistakes occur frequently in our daily lives, letters get lost in the mail, employers incorrectly record employee work hours, and new cars are recalled for mechanical defects. Likewise, physicians will also commit errors in their practice. We must accept, however, that our errors often have higher stakes in the sense that health has more meaning than material objects. In addition, because we do not practice medicine in an isolated vacuum, we must be concerned with not only our own mistakes but also the mistakes of others that are under our supervision.[4]

Even when there is no medical negligence performed, physicians may be scrutinized for the tough decisions that they are forced to make. These decisions are often made spontaneously in life or death situations, in situations where all data are not available, and in situations where there are many acceptable avenues from which to choose. As a consequence, the concept of retrospective criticism or 'Monday morning quarterbacking' has become popular in medical practices (i.e. morbidity and mortality conferences, quality and assurance meetings, etc.).[4]

Similarly, bad results sometimes occur even in the setting of the best medicine practiced. This concept is not well accepted by the plaintiff attorney community but is a natural consequence of life. Our lives do not proceed in perfection and we do not live in a utopia. Therefore, adverse outcomes are not necessarily the result of human error and are, therefore, sometimes inevitable.

Assure good turnover of patients at shift change

Without a doubt, shift change can be one of the most tumultuous times of the day in the emergency department or the private office. Incoming physicians and nurses take report from outgoing physicians and nurses. Delays in care are inevitable as reports are made and new providers become acquainted with the patients and their labs. Information that is relayed now becomes second and sometimes third-hand (e.g. emergency medical services report to first physician, then first physician reports to second physician). Orders may be postponed as secretaries also change. These multiple factors create a large crevice for potential errors to slip through.

Before losing faith and dreading the time of shift change, there are actions that can be implemented to make the switch more smoothly. At our hospital, we altered the physician change to 30 minutes prior to the nurse change. This has resulted in less confusion because the new doctor is already underway when the nurses are making their change. We also have nursing and physician shifts staggered so that there is always an overlap of nurses and physicians from different shifts.

As the physician signing out, always make sure that you discuss the patients that you are turning over directly with the physician accepting the patients. Give a 'bullet' presentation containing the pertinent points of the history, physical, and laboratory data. Then state what is pending and what your impression is at that time. We had one physician who would always take over 10 minutes to present each patient to us and then never be able to give us his impression. This was in essence a nuisance because we would spend 20–30 minutes getting check-out, fall three to four patients behind, and still be clueless as to the problems of the patients that we were inheriting. In the time that we spent on the check-out, we could have seen the patient ourselves. This defeats the purpose of the turnover of patients. Furthermore, it always helps the oncoming physician to have a feel of what you think the problem is. Finally, never sign out a pelvic or rectal exam to the next physician. Imagine the patient's image of the next physician when he or she walks in for the sole purpose of doing an intrusive exam on their body. The oncoming physician does not have the time to get as well acquainted as the first physician and should not be forced into this embarrassing position. In addition, you are taking a high risk that these exams that you defer will probably not get done. This practice would not be good medicine because you are not taking matters into your own hands.

After your sign-out is completed, make sure that you document on your chart the time you signed out the patient to the new physician. This is important because we read a case where the first physician treated a patient with chest pain and felt that the patient should have been admitted. He verbalized this to the second physician at sign-out but did not document it. The second physician discharged the patient once the labs were completed and the patient was found to have had an active myocardial infarction after discharge. Both emergency physicians were faulted for the inappropriate discharge since it was argued that the first physician did not discuss the patient with the second physician. Although it is not feasible to document the exact extent of your sign-out, a simple statement such as 'signed out to Dr Smith at 7 am' will keep the door open in the courtroom to elaborate on the extent of your sign-out. Omitting this simple statement, however, eliminates your opportunity to discuss your sign-out.

As the receiving physician, listen carefully to the check-out and ask your questions before the other physician leaves. Then assess among the patients already seen and the patients waiting to be seen the priority at which you will need to see them. Unless there are patients triaged as emergent, it is preferable to see the old patients first to make sure that they are stable and to organize your disposition plans and order more labs if needed. Otherwise, turnover patients sometimes stay in the ED for hours as they wait to be seen and new labs are ordered. Furthermore, because it has been repeatedly shown that many medical errors occur at check-out time, assume that the outgoing physician was not at his or her best during this time and evaluate the turnover patient to create your own impression.

Case 6.1 A faulty handoff

Edwards, in *The M & M Files*, presents a case where there was a poor turnover of a patient at shift change and this was coupled with a poor acceptance of the patient.[5] A 29-year-old man with a history of diabetes presented to the ED with weakness, nausea, and vomiting that all started after having nasal congestion and ear pain. He was found to be in diabetic ketoacidosis (DKA) with bilateral otitis media.

On presentation, he was slightly tachypneic and tachycardic. His blood work revealed glucose of 444 mg/dl, sodium of 131 mEq/L, and bicarbonate of 18 mEq/L. The ED physician called the on-call physician and recommended admission. The on-call physician, however, requested that the patient be treated in the ED and discharged if clinical status improved. The ED physician agreed and gave the patient insulin and fluids over three hours. She then signed the patient out to the next physician on duty.

The second ED physician repeated the blood work after the fluids were given. Although the glucose had improved to 355 mg/dl, the bicarbonate had only changed to 17 mEq/L. Since the patient was feeling better and was able to hold down fluids, he was discharged with an antibiotic for the treatment of otitis media.

The nausea and vomiting returned, however, as soon as the patient went home. Later that night, the man had a syncopal episode and suffered a

continued

forehead laceration. He returned to the ED and was admitted for four days. His primary physician questioned the medical director of the hospital why the patient was not admitted initially or why antiemetics were not prescribed.

This patient's emergency care was compromised in part because of the suboptimal turnover of his care between the two ED physicians. The initial physician was justified in believing that the patient needed to be admitted. Most, if not all, of the medical literature still recommends that all patients in DKA be admitted to the hospital. Although she agreed to treat the patient in the ED, this was only to see if the patient would show improvement. Because she was not around to make the disposition, she should have informed the oncoming physician that she wanted to admit this patient and that the on-call physician should be called for admission unless the patient showed dramatic improvement.

The oncoming physician did not accept the patient with full responsibility. He ordered repeat blood work that showed that the patient was still acidotic (actually worse) and did not admit him for this. He later claimed that the sign-out from the first physician was only that the patient was 'ready to roll' after a little more fluid and a quick recheck.[6] In essence, he was not serving as the patient's physician and rechecked his medical status, but he was merely 'babysitting' him before discharge.

Help your nurses prevent medication errors

Medication errors can occur anywhere along the chain from the order of the medication to the administration of the medication. We discuss in Chapter 8 some medication errors over which physicians have little control. In this section, we discuss how physicians and nurses can work together to decrease medication errors. A recent article by Cohen in *Nursing 2003* included a survey of nurses concerning medication errors generated some interesting tips.[7]

Periodically, inquire whether your nurses are following the 'five rights' of medication administration. The survey showed that 79% of nurses believed that most medication errors occur when a nurse carelessly neglects to follow the 'five rights' of medication administration.[8] These 'five rights' consist of right patient, right drug, right dose, right route, and right time. Our emergency nurse, Shirley Swanson, informed us that the sixth right is the patient's right to refuse. We invented the seventh right, 'write legibly.' The article gives an example of how Cerebyx can be misinterpreted as Celebrex if the handwriting is not clear.[9]

The survey also found that most nurses feel that oral orders (whether in person or via telephone) are more prone to errors than written orders.[10] Most nurses who responded to this survey stated that upon receiving an oral order, they write it directly on the patient's chart. They then read back the name of the drug, dose, and route to the prescriber.[11] This strategy serves as a check system for administrating the right medication. This policy recently became a JCAHO recommendation in its 2003 National Patient Safety Goals.[11]

The last tip from this article that we found helpful to implement among our nurses is to have them check for patient allergies before drug administration. Most nurses admitted to checking for allergies by asking the patient, and by checking the chart, ID bracelet, or MAR (medication administration record).[12] We cannot count the number of times that our nurses have prevented the inadvertent administration of an allergic medicine by double-checking with the patient.

Avoid decimal points and unnecessary zeros where they are not needed. They may create confusion or misunderstanding for the nurse that is going to administer the drug. Rarely, if ever, do you need to end a number with a decimal point and a zero (i.e. 6.0). It serves no useful purpose and may only be misinterpreted as 60. The following is a clinical example of this mistake.

Case 6.2 Look before you give

This example, from Selbst and Korin's *Preventing Malpractice Lawsuits in Pediatric Emergency Medicine*, is an unfortunate case of a preventable medication error.[13] After an infant was born by cesarean section due to suspected placental abruption, she was placed on mechanical ventilation and developed a Streptococcus pneumoniae infection. The neonatologist instructed the resident to administer vancomycin for the infant. The resident meant to write '35.0 mg' and the first nurse transferred the number correctly to the cardex. The second nurse, however, did not see the decimal point and gave the infant two doses of 350 mg of vancomycin. The child subsequently developed deafness and a lawsuit was filed against the neonatologist, the resident, the two nurses, and the hospital.

Help yourself prevent medication errors

Doherty, Segal, and McKinney wrote an article in the peer-review journal *Consultant* that specifically discusses the topic of prescription errors.[14] This article cites that medication errors are responsible for the death of up to 98 000 patients annually. It also focuses on errors that occur in the drug-prescribing stage. In other words, these are physician errors and not that of the nurses or pharmacists.

The first type of physician drug error arises when there is a lack of knowledge about the drug.[15] This lack of knowledge may cause errors in several ways. Drugs may be used without respect to their proper indications and contraindications. Within these two categories, there are further subdivisions into underuse, overuse, and misuse. Underuse is the failure to use a drug in a situation where it has shown to be of proven benefit to the patient. The example given is that of the angiotensin-converting enzyme (ACE) inhibitors or the angiotensin II receptor blockers to prevent the progression of diabetic nephropathy in a diabetic who has microalbuminuria. The same can be said for these medications for the patient with congestive heart failure to also prevent its progression.

Overuse occurs when there is the utilization of medications that are not necessary for a particular situation. An example is using the fluoroquinolone (broad-spectrum) antibiotics for uncomplicated infections, which are probably viral. This excessive treatment is harmful to the patient by creating resistance to powerful antibiotics that may be needed for future infections that are more serious. A variant form of overuse is treating a side effect of another medication without withdrawing that medication first. Examples here would include starting a diuretic for dependent leg edema that was caused by amlodipine or prescribing a cough medicine for a patient on an ACE inhibitor.

Misuse occurs when a medication is used inappropriately. The most common form of misuse is prescribing a medication that is contraindicated for a particular patient. Examples cited in the article include the prescription of amoxicillin for a patient with a penicillin allergy and prescribing metformin for a woman whose creatinine is greater than 1.4 mg/dl. Another common example is the prescription of pain medicines that contain Tylenol (Lortab) for patients with liver disease.

Another type of drug error resulting from lack of physician knowledge is that of dosing errors.[16] The authors of the article state that these errors tend to occur in the elderly when medications are started at moderate doses and not titrated up from low doses. The elderly are much more sensitive to changes in their physiology and the classic example of this is the development of orthostatic hypotension with moderate doses of blood pressure medications. We add two further types of dosing errors. The first is the underdosing of medications. For example, metronidazole is often used for vaginal and pelvic infections as 500 mg twice a day. This regimen, however, is inadequate for the treatment of diverticulitis, where the correct dosing is 500 mg four times a day. The second type of dosing error is prescribing the incorrect length of therapy. Typical examples are found in the treatment of chronic sinusitis and prostatitis. Both of these infections require prolonged (few to several weeks) courses of antibiotics and are not adequately treated with regimens used for acute sinusitis and urinary tract infections, respectively.

The final type of drug error from lack of physician knowledge is that of drug–drug interactions.[17] These types of error can sometimes be very occult and unanticipated by the physician. Interactions may occur with something else that the patient is taking or something else that the patient is eating. The physician may not be aware of these other ingestants. Over-the-counter cold remedies and alternative medicines are notorious for containing compounds that will interact with prescription medications. Certain foods and many drugs will have effects on the efficacy of warfarin metabolism. Finally, alcohol taken in combination with metronidazole will produce a disulfiram-like reaction.

The second type of physician drug error stems from a lack of patient information.[18] These can be subdivided into two main categories, those from inadequate records, and those from undocumented allergies. Inadequate records can become problematic anywhere in the continuum of patient care. The most commonplace is when the patient is hospitalized and the outpatient chart is incomplete with the proper medications and dosages.

Undocumented allergies are frequently problematic because patients tend to have a difficult time remembering drug names. We have seen charts where the patient states that they are allergic to 'an antibiotic' or 'a pain medicine.' It is easy to see the dilemma that the treating physician has if he or she obtains a chart with undocumented allergies in these types of patients. A subset of this group of errors from the lack of patient information is the case where intolerance or side effects are labeled as true allergies. Nausea and vomiting are side effects of many antibiotics and the listing of these medications as 'allergies' would severely narrow the physician's therapeutic choices.

The third type of physician drug error comes from communication failures.[19] Illegible handwriting, misunderstanding of verbal orders, and misinterpretation of abbreviations and decimals all represent communication failures. The authors suggest that physicians have the nurse or pharmacist who is taking their order repeat the order back to them for confirmation. They also cite that physicians are frequently guilty of not discussing adverse effects of medications with patients before prescribing them and not asking about side effects after they have been prescribed.

The final section of the article addresses drug errors that may occur in specific populations of patients. Children's medications are frequently weight-based and require correct computation. Make sure that there is no confusion whether the number written in the weight section represents pounds or kilograms. Some medications are not recommended in children because of its affect on bone growth (fluoroquinolones) or staining of teeth (tetracycline).

The elderly patient also requires special caution with the prescription of medications. Senior patients typically take multiple medications which predispose them to drug–drug interactions. As we discussed previously, their physiology is much more sensitive to small changes in medication dosages. Their ability to metabolize and excrete medications may be decreased due to declining renal function and nutritional status. Finally, they are much more susceptible to medication complications such as gastrointestinal bleeding, respiratory depression, and oversedation.

Sometimes you may avoid medicine errors in your practice by listening to the complaints of your patients. Patients frequently complain that another physician prescribed a medicine that was too expensive, that they were allergic to, that interacted with their other medicines, or gave them a deleterious effect. Whether you feel that their complaint has validity or not, it may give you insight into your own prescribing practices.

Case 6.3 Are the patient's medications compatible?

An example of such an instance occurred in our emergency department. A 62-year-old diabetic was brought to our facility by ambulance after his wife had found him confused and diaphoretic that morning. His blood sugar was 32 mg/dl when the paramedics arrived and checked it. He became more responsive after they gave him an ampule of intravenous 50% dextrose solution.

Upon his arrival to the ED, he was confused again and his repeat blood sugar was 44 mg/dl. After receiving 1 mg of intravenous glucagon and another ampule of intravenous 50% dextrose solution, he became alert again. He told us that he went to his private physician four days ago for an infection on his elbow and was placed on an antibiotic by the nurse practitioner but was otherwise feeling fine. He had no other recent illnesses or changes in medications or diet before his blood sugars started dropping

continued

that morning. He had normal vital signs and did not appear septic. This made us suspicious as to which antibiotic he was given.

After he told us it was a fluoroquinolone class of antibiotic, we informed him that this class of drugs has resulted in unpredictable blood sugars for some patients. (Although when we asked this question to pharmaceutical managers and their clinical experts, they are not all in agreement as to whether this unpredictability of blood sugars while taking a fluoroquinolone was a class effect or only from one particular fluoroquinolone.) We also told him that the elbow infection could be causing his sugars to fluctuate.

When the patient's primary physician came to admit the patient, he also told him that he believed that the hypoglycemic episode was probably due to the antibiotic. The patient and his wife became angry at the nurse practitioner. The patient told us that his good friend was a plaintiff attorney and that he was going to file a case against the nurse practitioner. The patient stated that 'she told me to check my temperatures several times a day, but she should have told me to check my blood sugars several times a day.' This statement was certainly food for thought for our own infectious management of diabetics.

Interestingly, we have used fluoroquinolones in diabetic patients for years with outstanding results. They have broad coverage for the polymicrobial infections that diabetics tend to acquire and are an excellent option for diabetics with skin infections who are allergic to penicillin drugs, as was the case with this patient. However, we will remember from this case that patients should be warned about the potential of fluctuating blood sugars when these antibiotics are used.

Be well read and trained

Medicine is a constantly evolving field and to practice good medicine, the physician must keep up with the current literature and skills. She can accomplish this through continuing medical education conferences, medical journals and books, and internet sites through her professional organization. Furthermore, there are ample opportunities for medical lectures through hospitals (grand rounds), through sales pharmaceuticals (dinner talks or teleconferences), and through CD-ROMs.

Medical skills should be periodically updated to maintain competency and to be aware of new developments. We recommend keeping certifications such as Advanced Cardiac Life Support (ACLS) up to date, even though you may not have had to use them since medical school. A good example that we use for this recommendation is that you never know when someone could have an anaphylactic reaction to a medication given in the office and require immediate treatment. A primary care colleague of ours told us that he does not keep his ACLS certification updated because he does not have a code cart in his office. How would he respond in court if a plaintiff attorney asked him if he thought that an anaphylactic reaction in the office was not possible? In addition, there are other skills taught in ACLS (e.g. Heimlich maneuver) that do not require a code cart.

Medical literature is continuously changing and updated. Standard medical references are generally updated every four years and even within that time frame, material can sometimes be outdated. Be careful about using outdated textbooks as references because they cannot be relied on to assist you in court should the treatment recommendations change. Furthermore, with the wealth of medical information (including text) in the internet and on CD-ROM, it becomes more and more unacceptable for physicians to not have access to current literature.

Know your medical terms

As a corollary to the preceding section, this section may seem simple but is equally important. Many physicians use preprinted medical forms that may contain specific medical terms. In addition, the medical language is fraught with terms that are given specific names (e.g. Murphy's sign, Homan's sign, etc.). Consequently, our charts may sometimes appear like a foreign language to non-medical reviewers.

With this in mind, if you are involved in a lawsuit, chances are good that a lawyer will ask you define these terms (sometimes in a courtroom in front of the jury). It would not only be embarrassing if you could not define them but also could be damaging to your case if you appear incompetent to the jury. For example, most physicians like to check the little box that states cranial nerves two through twelve are intact and normal. However, some of these physicians will have a difficult time responding if a lawyer should ask 'Can you explain doctor how you tested each cranial nerve?' Alternatively, he or she may ask, 'What constitutes a positive Homan's sign?'

A clinical example is the frequent diagnosis of hyperemesis gravidarum by emergency physicians. Almost every pregnant patient that is seen for nausea and vomiting receives this diagnosis once other medical etiologies are ruled out. The term 'hyperemesis gravidarum', however, applies to a restricted group of patients with vomiting in pregnancy. The criteria for this diagnosis require at least one of the following: abnormal electrolytes, weight loss greater than 5% of prepregnancy weight, or ketonemia.[20] Otherwise, the diagnosis is nausea and vomiting of pregnancy. We are not sure if the clinical management of the two is any different but using correct terminology avoids scrutiny of your knowledge.

The gist of this section is to make sure that you are familiar with your medical terms in your documentation. We all learned these terms in medical school and sometimes we continue to use them gratuitously and forget the significance they carry. For the most part, these fine details do no make a clinical difference in treating the patient. However, remember that the goal of plaintiff attorneys is to make you look incompetent, either in the deposition or in court. Therefore, even though you may have forgotten some of the details of the medical terms that you use, make sure that you do your homework before attending a deposition or a trial.

Do not give the impression that you work for the pharmaceutical companies

In the same manner as any other business, pharmaceutical companies have tried numerous methods of attracting physicians to their product. They will print their product insignia on just about any product that you can imagine and give it to physicians in order to advertise their product. This includes preprinted prescriptions, progress notes, laboratory coats, scrubs, etc. We have all seen many of our colleagues use these products in their daily practice.

At the 2003 American Academy of Family Physicians Scientific Assembly, we attended a lecture by Edward Zurad MD. Dr Zurad gave a brilliant lecture on 'Reducing Malpractice Errors.' In his talk, he encouraged physicians never to give the impression that they are working for the pharmaceutical companies. He gave the example of physicians who use progress notes preprinted with drug insignia on them. He presented the scenario of having these notes magnified 10 times and shown to a jury in court and proposed that the jury would not have a good impression of the physician if they thought the physician could be influenced by a particular drug company. We agree with his comment and would add that patients would not feel comfortable that their physician is prescribing the best medicines for them if they see that physician wearing a drug-sponsored laboratory coat or scrub. Although some physicians may not agree with the above comments, our encouragement is that as a professional, you should try to stay as neutral as possible.

Develop 'standards of practice'

Dr Zurad also encouraged physicians to develop a 'standard of practice' in their office. He defined 'standard of practice' as routines that you carry out with every patient without deviation. Examples from his practice include discussing all the side effects and interactions of any new medications that he prescribes and utilizing a female chaperone for every breast or pelvic examination. 'Standards of practice' serve as a reminder for him to consistently perform certain routines in his practice. Although he does not routinely dictate these practices in his notes, he is without doubt if a plaintiff attorney ever questions him about these practices. He offered a great quote on this subject: 'try to make as many things in your practice as black and white as possible, no gray zones.'

Again, we feel that his advice is wise and helpful. First, it maintains a constant level of care that should not be breached. Second, because it is not feasible to dictate these practices in every patient's notes, you can have your nursing staff or other patients confirm your standards if they have witnessed them routinely. Finally, you will feel much more confident and assured during questioning at interrogatories, deposition, and in court.

You must consistently comply with your 'standards of practice', however. If you do not, your staff will be the first to notice and will not be able to concur with your story in court. In addition, you may become confused and inconsistent in telling the judge and jurors about the events in question if you were not consistent.

Physicians should address non-emergent but potentially serious problems

Physicians frequently order routine tests in the office or the emergency department. These include blood work, X-rays, urinalysis, cultures, etc. Some of the results of these tests are not immediately available and the treating physician frequently has to make a preliminary interpretation. The prime example is that of X-rays, where most centers do not have the radiologist give official interpretation until one to two days later. These official readings will often be more complete and contain non-emergent details that urgent care physicians and emergency physicians may not look for.

Case 6.4 There are no small details

Dr Zurad gave a case in Pennsylvania that is similar to many that we have come across in our practice. A man treated for pneumonia at an emergency department in Pennsylvania had a formal chest X-ray reading of a pulmonary nodule. The man recovered from the pneumonia but was never informed of this nodule. Shortly later, he suffered complications from lung cancer and sued the emergency physician. The case was settled for $1.25 million.

Although emergency physicians can argue that pulmonary nodules are not within the scope of emergency medicine and it should not be their responsibility for following non-emergent problems, they should still always remember what constitutes good medicine. Good medicine consists of treating patients as if they were our own family members. We must ask ourselves the question, 'If this patient were my mother or father, would I want them to know this information?' Treating, in this case, is as simple as informing the patient and making an appropriate referral.

Be careful about prescribing medicines to a patient without examining them

We were hesitant about including this section in the book because it would make many physicians and many patients upset. Phone medicine and treatment has long been a convenient method for people to give and receive medical care that is also cost-efficient for the healthcare industry. The physician is happy, the patient is happy, the emergency department is happy because they do not have to see the patient during off hours, and money is saved. So why are we recommending against it?

When we were in residency, a heated debate existed annually regarding which residents should be allowed to do phone triage. The senior residents always wanted to pass the duties to the interns. However, the attending physicians were always resistant to letting this happen because of the medical liability that was involved. One attending stated that 'phone medicine is much more difficult than office medicine.' This belief was shared by most of the other attending physicians and numerous factors contribute to this belief.

Phone medicine deprives the physician of the second most important part of the medical evaluation – the physical exam (the first being the history). Without seeing and examining the patient, you cannot obtain the subtle nuances that are usually present with observation of the patient. You cannot confirm the patient's history with a physical exam or determine key physical findings that may not be part of the patient's history. Furthermore, when patients are poor historians and/or one does not have the patient's chart at his or her access, there can be compromise in good medical care.

We feel that the most important argument against phone medicine is that it is extremely difficult to defend in court. Just imagine a plaintiff attorney asking, 'How can you prescribe medicine to a patient you never saw?' or 'How can you think you could treat this patient without examining the patient?' We have all heard the arguments against internet pharmacies prescribing medicines and internet physicians treating patients without seeing them. Most of these same arguments could be used against phone medicine. The only difference is that there may be a prior relationship between the physician and the patient. By default, phone medicine cannot lead to good documentation because of its incompleteness.

The most common example of phone medicine is the prescribing of antibiotics for infectious symptoms. Specifically, pediatric patients are routinely called in antibiotics for 'ear infections' over the phone. We feel that this is a dangerous practice habit as we have seen many of the missed diagnoses in our emergency department (e.g. pneumonia, meningitis). Furthermore, fever and infections in children represent some of the most common malpractice suits and also some of the biggest payout types of suits in pediatric practice. Our experience has taught us that a febrile child is usually more difficult to evaluate in person than an adult due to atypical symptoms and limited history. Therefore, we can only imagine how much more difficult it would be to evaluate through telephone conversation only.

Without physically seeing and examining a patient, false assumptions may occasionally be made concerning the patient's diagnosis. This may lead to improper medications or instructions given to the patient.

Case 6.5 Long-distance medicine

The following is an excellent example from Selbst and Korin's *Preventing Malpractice Lawsuits in Pediatric Emergency Medicine*.[21] Although this patient was not treated over the phone, he was treated from a distance without an actual examination. A teenager was brought into the ED with an 'asthma' attack. The physician on duty had treated about 20 similar patients on that shift with epinephrine with good response. Hence, looking at the child from a distance, he ordered the nurse to give this child an injection of epinephrine. A chest X-ray taken after the injection was given showed cardiomegaly. The patient was also found to be hypertensive and had urine that was tea-colored. The patient had glomerulonephritis with the

continued

secondary complications of hypertension and congestive heart failure and did not have asthma. Because the patient was relatively young, the epinephrine did not cause any harm. The outcome would most certainly have been different had the patient been older with more advanced cardiovascular disease. The administration of epinephrine was preventable had the patient taken the time to perform a quick examination of the patient.

Serve as a good citizen

Like it or not, as a physician, you are a public figure. Your image and reputation is constantly under scrutiny and observation from the public, your colleagues, your co-workers, hospital or clinic administrators, and state health agencies. In fact, the entire concept of 'being a good physician' includes the maintenance of a commendable reputation. This is true in all professional occupations (e.g. physicians, lawyers, legislators, etc.).

Although physicians enjoy diverse activities and have varied personalities just like members of any other profession, our professional appearance and manners are typically expected by the public to be of a conservative nature. We have noticed through the years that when physicians harbor behaviors that are not represented by the majority of other physicians (e.g. males with earrings, tattoos, tobacco use, alcoholic tendencies, etc.), rumors or statements of reputations spread quickly among patients, staff, and other physicians. Remember that in our profession, we never know whom we will meet on a given day. On the day that we may not look or act our best, we may interact with our future judges or jurors.

Physicians also need to be careful in their private lives concerning brushes with the law because these interactions will likely be broadcast to others either through media or through rumors. Convictions of arrest, driving while intoxicated, sexual harassment, domestic violence, etc. are likely to injure a physician's career when others begin to lose trust in the physician. We remember reading a front-page article in our local paper about a prominent attorney who was in a hurry to catch a plane after a long day at the office. He forgot to remove or report his revolver from his suitcase and had it detected by the metal detector at the airport. He was arrested and received very negative publicity in the local paper. Remember that if you have any brushes with the law, these incidents will surely be emphasized in any malpractice suit against you (through interrogatories, deposition, etc.).

We would like to give a special mention of the alcohol problem in the medical profession. When we were in medical school, we were told that physicians had one of the highest rates of alcohol abuse of any profession. Indeed, physicians have many opportunities for alcohol consumption through the numerous dinners and meetings that we are invited to. We are not even mild alcohol drinkers but we try to not consume any alcohol eight hours before we have to perform medical work in any form. This is because even one drink will leave alcohol on your breath, which can create unwanted impressions to your patients, staff, and colleagues. While we were in our last year of residency, we were given permission from our chief resident to leave hospital coverage for one hour for an end-of-year party. The stipulation was that no alcohol could be consumed. We complied by this rule and did not partake of any alcohol. However, as soon as we returned to duty, the chief resident grabbed our shirt and pulled us up to his nose in order for him to smell our breath. We created the eight-hour rule because we feel that we owe it to our patients to not be impaired.

Give returning patients a step-up in evaluation

The patient who returns, to the emergency department or to the office, because he is not feeling better is referred to as the 'bounce-back' patient. While the physician may be tempted to develop an initial frustration that this patient has returned and requires another evaluation, she should regard this as a golden opportunity 'to make things better.' The patient has trusted you or your colleagues enough to return to your care. This is much better than the patient that worsens but does not return or goes somewhere else where they may be deteriorating. You may discover the patient's complications from a subsequent complaint and/or lawsuit.

Keep in mind that most 'bounce-back' patients will require a step-up in evaluation. Although some will return with new manifestations or have their previous labs change significantly to make the diagnosis clearer, most will necessitate a more extensive evaluation than that provided in the first visit. This can come in the form of getting a consultant involved, ordering additional tests, observing the patient for a longer period, or administering a different medication to the patient. This shows that the physician is actively entertaining new considerations for the patient's clinical problem. Previous charts and tests should be obtained and their review documented in the chart.

If the patient is still not better after your second evaluation, you should strongly consider admitting the patient or referring to specialty care if possible. A plaintiff attorney's eyes will widen when they see multiple visits and discharge without improvement, particularly when step-up in evaluations were not performed on subsequent visits.

Case 6.6 Take advantage of second opportunities

Edwards describes the consequences of failing to give a step-up in care through a case in *The M & M Files*.[22] A 19-year-old Hispanic male presented to the ED complaining of chest pain and numbness in his left arm. The pain was pleuritic and had been present for the past 24 hours. He appeared anxious on exam and was tachycardic with a pulse of 105 beats/minute. The ED physician ordered a chest X-ray, which was normal, and discharged the patient with 'possible pleurisy' and gave him a dose of ibuprofen.

The patient returned to the ED the following day with the same complaint and saw a different ED physician. The patient again appeared anxious and was tachycardic with a pulse of 105 beats/minute. After reviewing the chart from the previous day, the second physician ordered a complete blood count. The test was normal and the patient was discharged with the diagnoses of anxiety and atypical chest pain.

continued

The next day prompted a third visit to the ED. He was still complaining of chest pain and had the same elevated pulse. The third ED physician to see this patient ordered an electrocardiogram (EKG), which showed a sinus tachycardia and changes consistent with early repolarization. He also ordered a chest X-ray, which was again normal. The physician, however, noted that the patient was in extreme discomfort and gave him a prescription for lorazepam and discharged him.

The patient made a fourth visit to the ED that evening and saw the first ED physician again. The physician became outraged and pulled the patient's family aside and told them that the patient was too young to have cardiac disease and that they were accumulating excessive medical expenses and should follow up with his primary physician. After the family stated that they could not get the patient an appointment with his physician for a week, the ED physician gave them an alternate physician to follow up with and discharged the patient.

The patient was admitted to a different hospital three days later with the diagnosis of viral myocarditis. The patient's clinical state had severely worsened by this time. The ED director from the admitting hospital complained to the ED director from the first hospital that the diagnosis of myocarditis was inexcusably missed during four visits to the emergency department.

In his discussion of this case, Edwards points out that each ED physician bought into the diagnosis of the first ED physician during the patient's three subsequent visits to the department. Instead of considering anxiety as the traditional diagnosis of exclusion in the evaluation of chest pain, they made it the diagnosis of inclusion. This mode of thinking prevented them from entertaining the correct diagnosis. Edwards advises, you should 'approach the return-visit patients with a fresh perspective and assume that something may have been missed.'[23]

Be proud and supportive of your profession

Although most, if not all, of us have been affected by the current medical malpractice crisis (getting sued, losing insurance carrier, not being able to afford insurance, etc.), we must continue to practice medicine with the dignity and professionalism that we were taught in medical school. As reported in a survey of the public in *AMA News* in 2002, we are still the most respected profession in the United States and there are still thousands of young bright college students that aspire to be able to do what we do. We cannot display negativity to these young promising adults and discourage them from entering our field because we may need them to take care of our loved ones and us in the future.

We had the opportunity for several years to work with the State of Florida Department of Health in creating the Florida Medical Licensure Exam. This exam was given to foreign medical graduates in order to certify them to practice under the supervision of a licensed physician in the State of Florida. The test was administered twice a year for over two years and the typical passing percentage was less than 1%. As members of the committee who wrote, reviewed, and edited the questions, we did not feel that the test was much different in degree of difficulty from the United States Medical Licensure Exam Step 3 that all American medical residents take to obtain their license. Our experience on this committee convinced us that American trained physicians are still one of the best educated groups of physicians in the world. Therefore, we should not take belief in the negative press and comments from plaintiff attorneys stating that there are 'too many bad doctors out there.' It is simply not true.

Our profession has always been and remains one of the most active and generous professions in the community. In almost every city across the United States, there are free clinics staffed with physicians who volunteer their time and energy. Some physicians also provide on-site free medical care through their church groups (to migrant workers). American physicians have always been extremely active in giving their time and skills to help third-world countries through missionary trips. Finally, we are a profession that provides our skills to people that emergently need it 24 hours a day, every day of the year regardless of the recipient's ability to pay (in many facilities in the United States the no-pay percentage may range as high as 70–80%). Physicians should not let these numbers discourage them; rather, we should let them affirm our vital role in society. There are very few other professions, if any, in the United States that can make these statements.

Our profession places us in a great position; one where we are able to make a difference in people's lives every day. That is something that we must be proud of and fulfill to the best of our ability. We feel that pride gives one the energy to perform one's best and, subsequently, decreases the opportunity for error. Indeed, this has been our feeling during the times that we have taken a break from our regular jobs to volunteer our services to the community.

Assume your chart documentation will be read by others

As discussed in the introduction, this statement is not to emphasize paranoia. Rather, it is to remind you that we are public figures whose actions are reviewed by many. It also serves to remind you of the legal climate in which we currently live. As one of the fundamentals lesson of medicine, preventing damage with primary prevention is a lot easier than controlling damage with secondary prevention. There is very little that you can do once a lawsuit is filed, so be certain your treatment and documentation of the case is thorough (and do not even give any thought of altering or destroying records). Remember that the foundation of any good defense (e.g. sports, combat, medicine, etc.) is anticipation.

Keeping the above mindset will prevent you from inserting derogatory or judgmental statements into the medical record. In turn, your medical decisions are likely to be more objective and in the best interest of the patient. You will also develop the habit of paying meticulous attention to clues and details from the patient's history and physical exam. Furthermore, considering the thoughts of an expert witness (playing devil's advocate) in your decision making will force you to expand on your medical reasoning. The net result of all this is that the medical care will be improved and less likely to undergo scrutiny.

Never believe that you are immune from legal action. As we have discussed in other chapters of this book, even the best doctors get sued. We are certainly not perfect individuals who are incapable of error, and even if we were, there is much in medicine that is beyond our control. Therefore, practice defensive medicine and take control of what you can. Remember that primary prevention is a lot easier and less stressful than defending oneself once a suit has been filed.

Case 6.7 Protecting yourself from criticism

Edwards provides an excellent case in *The M & M Files*.[24] An 82-year-old woman visited her primary physician for a headache and was found to have a subdural hematoma on CT scan. She had been having headaches for four weeks since she had an incident where she stumbled in a hallway and hit her head. On that occasion, she was brought to the emergency department where she was evaluated and discharged without any radiologic test. Her son, who is an attorney, called the hospital and complained about his mother's treatment in the ED.

The ED medical director reviewed the case and was satisfied with the medical care that his physician had given the patient based on his excellent documentation. The physician noted that the 'fall had been caused by a brief sense of imbalance when the patient turned a corner...and such sensations in similar circumstances were common for her.'[25] He wrote that there was no syncope or loss of consciousness and the patient did not have any neck tenderness. Furthermore, he recorded that the patient was not taking any anticoagulants and had a normal neurologic exam that did not change during her stay in the ED. Specific and clear discharge and follow-up instructions were given to the patient. The medical director concluded that this detailed and excellent documentation justified the medical care that was given and supported the decision of the treating physician against ordering a CT scan. From this example, we can see that adverse outcomes are much easier to defend if we anticipate that are charts will be reviewed. Had the emergency physician performed the same detailed evaluation but failed to document it, this case probably would have resulted in a successful lawsuit for the plaintiff.

Complete your medical notes and documents in a timely fashion

Much of what was said in the previous paragraphs also applies here. Most of us are very thorough at obtaining a history and performing a physical exam. However, during our busy practice, we sometimes will see and treat multiple patients before we get a chance to sit down and do our documentation. On occasion, this sit down period will come at the conclusion of the day when there are over 20 charts that need to be dictated.

We believe that each patient encounter has a standardized portion and an individualized portion. The standardized portion is the same for any patient that presents with a similar complaint and can usually be dictated or transcribed at a later time without sacrificing details. The individualized portion, however, is unique to each patient and an essential component of defensive medicine. The physician's input in this portion shows that he or she considered the patient's specific situation and this input could make the difference between a successful and unsuccessful defense. Therefore, delays in transcribing or dictating your patient encounter places the important, fine details of the individualized portion at risk for omission. There is much legal truth in the statement 'if it isn't in the chart, you didn't do it.'

The last issue on this topic has to deal with signing your charts. We frequently give verbal orders or standing orders to nurses. These orders are not signed immediately. Dictations are another example of chart documents that require a signature at a later date. Make sure that you sign and complete all of your required documentation in a prompt manner. If a document is reviewed that is not signed, the reviewers may develop a careless and lackadaisical impression of the physician. In addition, signing charts in a prompt fashion increases your memories of the encounters. This will enable you to make any necessary corrections to the dictations.

Develop peer review of charts in your practice

There are two clichés that are worth remembering in medicine: 'no-one is perfect'; and 'two heads are better than one.' All physicians will, on occasion, make treatment decisions that seem to deviate from the standard of care. It may happen from lack of experience, mental distraction from personal problems, or something that we just did not pick up on during our evaluation. These occasions are not only more likely to lead to adverse outcomes, but they are also more likely to lead to poor documentation. Therefore, some hospital practices have developed policies for having peer review of selected charts. Examples of selection criteria for peer reviews may be all pneumonia cases, all myocardial infarction cases, cases where the patient leaves against medical advice, every tenth case, etc.

Having a colleague review a case will sometimes lead to the detection of medical care that is considered 'substandard.' This is because a reviewer is not emotionally attached to the case and is able to review it objectively as it is documented.

Case 6.8 Two heads are better than one

Edwards has a good example of the benefits of such a program in *The M & M Files*.[26] He writes about one emergency department that installed a policy for peer reviewing every fourth chart. On the first day that the program was installed, the case of a 29-year-old woman who came to the ED for a headache the previous day was reviewed. The treating physician noted that the patient had a sudden development of a headache while she was taking a shower and that she had no prior history of headaches. Furthermore, her pain was most severe at the initial onset. He recorded a normal neurologic exam, then gave her an analgesic and discharged her with a diagnosis of 'acute cephalgia.'

continued

The reviewing physician became alarmed that the events noted in the chart were consistent with the classical findings of a subarachnoid hemorrhage. She immediately called the patient and asked her to return to the ED for further evaluation. This included a head CT, which did not show a hemorrhage and a lumbar puncture, which showed an abnormal number of red blood cells and slight xanthochromia. These findings were consistent with those of a subarachnoid hemorrhage. The patient did well after having a brain artery aneurysm clipped. Edwards points out that the treating ED physician 'was a per-diem moonlighter with an internal medicine background who was relatively new to emergency medicine.'[27] Therefore, this physician was 'not perfect' due to his inexperience.

Be your worst critic

Constantly evaluate and re-evaluate yourself as a physician. Consider whether you are giving each patient the best medical care that you are capable of. Are you treating each patient as if he is your own family member? Are you following recommended guidelines that are in current and standardized references for your specialty? (These are the guidelines by which plaintiff attorneys and expert witnesses expect you to abide.) How about practicing within the 'standard of care' within your community? If the answer to any of these questions is no, then you are not necessarily practicing bad medicine, but you are practicing high liability medicine.

Set the highest standards for your medical practice. Evaluate patients in a similar manner regardless of their age, race, sex, or financial status. We are not advocating a shopping spree with diagnostic tests for the self-paying patient. However, we explain to every patient with a suspected condition the test that we would recommend for that condition. If the patient then objects to the test based on financial concerns, we make sure that they understand any possible risks and offer them any possible alternative, albeit less optimal, test that may be available. The goal is to recommend the best possible test and let the patient make an educated decision. Furthermore, do not let personal factors affect how you evaluate a patient. A patient should receive the same evaluation at 2 am as they would at 10 am. Do not let personal problems with your own life (working too many hours, argument with family, etc.) interfere with your professional relationship with a patient. Finally, take careful consideration of any patient complaint that you receive and determine if you need to make any changes to your practice. Remember, a complaint may sometimes be a precursor to legal action.

Utilize telephone follow-ups with your patients

This practice will decrease your medical liability in several ways. It gives you a chance to see how a patient you saw recently is doing. This is helpful for the patient for whom you may not have had a clear diagnosis or the patient that had a diagnosis that could potentially worsen. Telephone follow-up gives the physician an opportunity to direct further medical treatment, if necessary, and obtain more or new information that may not have been obtained during the office visit. Timely phone calls will decrease liability by averting or abating adverse outcomes. In addition, patients will sense an increased concern for their health from your follow-up call and an improved doctor–patient relationship will result. Furthermore, in cases where there is a bad outcome and litigation results, telephone follow-up conversations will add credibility to the physician's concern and dependability.

Respect other physicians

Sometimes, especially if you work in an emergency setting, you will be sent patients from another physician to evaluate. Often, these patients will arrive with a preliminary diagnosis from the referring physician. Upon your evaluation, even if you discover that the initial diagnosis is unlikely, you must thoroughly reconsider the private physician's diagnosis. Could he or she obtain something from the history that you did not? Could the patient's behavior at their primary physician's office have been different than it is now? Always remind yourself that the primary physician has two implicit advantages that you do not. First, the primary physician treats this patient regularly and knows this patient far better than you could hope to in 15–20 minutes. Second, the primary physician was able to witness the extremely important 'first impression' of the presenting problem. After thorough consideration of the above factors, even if you still feel strongly that the primary physician's diagnosis is inaccurate, you should still, most of the time, order any test or consultation that the primary physician requested. The reason is that the patient expects to have this test or consultation and you will have no defense from the patient or his or her primary doctor if an adverse outcome ensues (even if the adverse outcome may or may not have been detected with the test or consultation). Furthermore, an antagonistic relationship will develop between the patient and you (if you cannot firmly convince the patient of your diagnosis) and between the patient's primary physician and you. Remember that patients are more likely to trust the physician that has been treating them for years than the physician that will spend 15 minutes or less with them. In cases where we are 100% sure that the test is not needed (this is exceptionally rare), we will inform the patient that 'we do not believe that your diagnosis is this.' We then proceed to explain to them why we believe so. Finally, we add that 'we respect your physician's opinion and will order the test if you feel that you need it.' The caveat to using this technique is that you must explain to the patient the alternatives to doing the test (i.e. less invasive or expensive tests, more careful observation for worsening symptoms, etc.). Regardless of the approach that you use, you must be diplomatic when evaluating another physician's patient so that you are respectful and courteous to the patient and the patient's physician. Contrary behavior will be very damaging to your case should an adverse outcome lead to a lawsuit.

Case 6.9 Keeping an open mind

A 69-year-old female was referred to us in the ED to 'rule out meningitis.' The referring physician's note stated that the patient had a headache and stiff neck. The patient appeared in no acute distress and denied any fevers, confusion, vomiting, or recent illness. She did state that this was the worst headache of her life. Although she was able to move her neck in all directions, she had pain with neck flexion. The remainder of her neurologic exam was unremarkable. Her temperature was normal.

Our first impression was that this patient had a low likelihood for meningitis. She possessed only one of the three main criteria that we usually seek in meningitis (fever, neck stiffness, and confusion). We also knew the referring physician. Earlier in the week, she had diagnosed a 19-year-old female with a headache and a fever as having sinusitis. The patient saw us in the ED the following day and was found to have viral meningitis. Therefore, we felt that the physician might have been extra-cautious with this patient.

Our greater concern for this patient was to rule out subarachnoid hemorrhage. We informed the patient of our thoughts and recommended a lumbar puncture if her head CT was normal. We told her that meningitis was unlikely but the lumbar puncture should be able to rule this out. The patient's head CT was normal. The lumbar puncture, however, revealed cloudy fluid. The white cell count was 96 000 cells/microliter in tubes #1 and #3. Her cerebrospinal fluid glucose was extremely low while the protein was markedly elevated. She was admitted for bacterial meningitis and her cerebrospinal fluid culture eventually grew Streptococcus pneumoniae. She made an uneventful recovery. We were glad that we did not ignore the opinion of the referring physician. We probably would not have forgiven ourselves if we had missed this diagnosis. In addition, the patient and the referring physician would also probably not have forgiven us.

Make effective use of consultants

Medicine is a multi-faceted academic field with many different specialties and subspecialties. In dealing with illnesses that may pertain to an isolated field (e.g. cardiology, gastroenterology, orthopedics, etc.), it is often considered 'standard of care' to discuss the case with the respective specialist if you are unsure of the best treatment plan. In fact, even if you are sure, a documented conversation with the specialist and getting their approval of your plan will ultimately decrease your liability if your plan does not lead to good results. Furthermore, we find that discussions of patient cases serve as an opportunity to improve our knowledge base in that particular field, which would also decrease our medical liability in the future. Plaintiff attorneys love to use specialists as expert witnesses. Therefore, incorporating the help of a specialist in your treatment decisions may 'even the odds' in the event of a lawsuit.

Remember that medicine in the United States has become highly specialized and patients are well familiar with this concept. Some patients will expect that their problems be discussed with the respective specialist. Other patients will come to the emergency department knowing only the name of their specialist. They will not even know who their primary care provider is. Therefore, for these patients, it is often reassuring to let them know that their problem has been discussed with the specialist. In the event of a bad outcome, they will be more likely to believe that good medicine was still practiced.

Be well read on medical-legal cases and issues

Some of the publications we use are *Corlandt Forum*, *Medical Economics*, *EMpulse*, *Physicians Financial News*, *Florida Medical Business*, *Foresight* (a publication of the American College of Emergency Physicians), and *American Medical News*, but there are certainly many more in circulation. In addition, there are an increasing number of medical-legal books available today. Some that we particularly like are *Doctors and the Law*[28], *Preventing Malpractice Lawsuits in Pediatric Emergency Medicine*[29], *Law For Physicians: an overview of medical legal issues*[30], *The M & M Files: morbidity & mortality rounds in emergency medicine*[31], *Errors, Medicine and the Law*[32], *Legal Problems in Emergency Medicine*[33], and *Medical Malpractice: solving the crisis*[34]. We are firm believers in the adage 'learn from other people's mistakes.' Reading about the malpractice cases of your colleagues helps you understand the legal processes of a lawsuit, the emotions that are involved in a lawsuit, the 'standard of care' for certain medical issues, and the outcomes of cases. Most importantly, in our opinion, medical-legal literature gives us insight into the techniques and thought processes of plaintiff attorneys. We, as physicians, can also be better adept at serving our profession if we keep ourselves knowledgeable about the current malpractice reform legislation and stay active in the political field.

For those physicians who are fortunate enough to work at an academic teaching institution, we recommend that you attend the morbidity and mortality conferences. These provide an excellent opportunity to hear about and learn from cases with adverse outcomes involving physicians and patients. They also tend to generate discussions concerning the 'standard of care' within your own community. Finally, physicians will have the chance to observe the opinions of other hospital personnel such as risk management coordinators, hospital attorneys, nursing supervisors, etc.

Know about your medications

Although this task seems impractical with the myriad current drugs and the drugs on the horizon, there are a few methods that may make things easier. In our ED, we have preprinted sheets on the most common medications that we give to patients explaining side effects and interactions. You can also remind the patient to make sure they talk to the pharmacist or read the information from the pharmacy when they pick up their medicines. To stay current with the latest drugs reaching the market and the cost of drugs, we rely a lot on pharmaceutical sales representatives to give us this information. We know that some physicians feel differently about drug representatives in their office and an alternative for these physicians would be reading advertisements in medical journals that can give them similar information. The public (plaintiff attorneys and jurors included) expects us, as physicians, to be fully aware of the medicines that we prescribe. In the event of an adverse outcome due to the effects of taking or not taking a medicine, plaintiff attorneys will commonly ask physicians if they informed the patient how much a medicine cost or if they explained to the patient the possible side effects.

Having stated the comments in the preceding paragraph, we recommend that you try to minimize writing prescriptions unless you have the patient's chart in front of you. Patients will often call you on the phone or stop you in the hallway to ask for prescriptions. Sometimes, these requests may be for medications that the patient has never taken before or for a problem for which they have never seen you. You are at a distinct disadvantage if you do not have the patient's chart in front of you. You will not have access to their allergies, the other medications that they are taking, the type of insurance they have, etc.

Be careful when selecting partners for your practice

Plaintiff lawyers use a common practice when it comes to choosing whose name to place on a lawsuit. Generally, they will include as many names and as many corporations as possible with the hope that they will find financial liability from someone or something. We have all read about cases where a physician was named in a suit for a patient that he or she never took care of.

Case 6.10 Pick your partners wisely

One particular case we would like to make reference to is found in an article entitled 'Are you liable for a colleague's mistake?' from the June 2003 *Medical Economics* journal.[35] In this article, a physician was named in a lawsuit of another physician's misdiagnosis because the physician had shared an office space with the physician at fault. Although the two physicians were not partners or employees of each other, the suit was filed under the theory of apparent or 'ostensible agency.' Despite the physician not at fault being eventually dismissed from this suit, it is easy to see how careless choices of partners can land your name in a lawsuit.

Case 6.11 Physicians who 'cherry-pick'

We worked with a partner early in our careers who had a habit of choosing the patients that he would like to see. He would skim over all the charts that were in the rack and choose those of young females. Then, he would proceed to spend excessive time evaluating his chosen patients. We are glad to say that he did not last very long in our practice because of the legal and ethical dilemmas that his style of practice created. Triaging patients by their demographics is not only ethically wrong; it is also medically unjustifiable and not consistent with the Hippocratic Oath of 'doing no harm.' He was not helping and (potentially harming) those that needed help first.

Be careful when selecting employees for your practice

As we discussed above, the physician is often responsible for other medical personnel in the practice. This includes nursing, medical assistants, secretaries, and sometimes laboratory and radiology technicians. Remember that we are considered the 'deep pocket' and therefore any legal action is likely to be targeted at us. Furthermore, patients perceive that the physician is ultimately responsible for the actions of others in the office or the emergency department.

Horn *et al.* recommend that a formal and efficient disciplinary policy be installed for each medical practice. These policies will become useful in the event that accusations of misconduct against medical staff result in legal action. However, they also point out that a disciplinary file can be a double-edged sword. If a file fails to record some incidents, the opposing attorney will interpret this as 'hiding the truth' or lack of supervision.[36] In contrast, if a file contains multiple records of incidents, the opposing attorney will question the physician's ability to take corrective action.

In general, Horn *et al.* recommend maintaining a disciplinary profile that includes the following:

1 A standardized, documented, periodic review of all employees.
2 A procedure by which errors or incidents are recorded, addressed, and remedied with employees.
3 Finally, full documentation of all disciplinary actions.[37]

They feel that any policy with the above stipulations would not only minimize the amount of medical errors committed by medical staff but also help convince to the courts that the physician is 'making every effort to maintain a competent and careful staff and should not be held responsible for a particular employee's actions.'[37]

Follow treatment guidelines and protocols

Whenever there is a malpractice lawsuit, the plaintiff attorney tries to prove that the standard of care is broken and the adverse outcome is the result of it. That is why treatment protocols are often the ace in the hole for plaintiff attorneys. In fact, we were at a meeting with the regional manager of Aventis recently discussing the product Lovenox and its use in Venous Thromboembolism (VTE) prophylaxis. He commented that more trial lawyers ordered the 2001 American College of Chest Physicians guidelines for VTE prophylaxis than any other group (including physicians). Having said this, you can assume that if there are established printed guidelines for medical management of a particular problem, the plaintiff attorney will be very familiar with them.

As physicians, most of us (if not all) will attest that adverse outcomes will arise in some situations despite appropriate medical care per established protocols. However, the efficacies of protocols are established through clinical studies because of their proven low morbidity and mortality. Therefore, poor outcomes are much easier to defend when protocols are followed than outcomes that result from medical treatment that does not follow the 'standard of care.' Despite the fact that most physicians are probably aware of the availability of treatment protocols, three recent articles suggest that not enough of us are following them.

In a recent study on lipid management in elderly patients, it was found that cholesterol therapy was given to approximately 50% of patients with a history of myocardial infarction, 41–46% of patients with a history of stroke, and 40–50% of patients with peripheral arterial disease. Nass states that 'this pattern of undertreatment is consistent with findings from samples of adults of all ages with known vascular disease.'[38] The CRUSADE (Can Rapid risk stratification of Unstable angina patients Suppress ADverse outcomes with Early implementation) study showed that aspirin was used in 90% of patients, beta-blockers in 76% of patients, heparin in 83% of patients, GP IIb-IIIa in 31% of patients, and clopidogrel (Plavix) in 35% of patients.[39] Another article demonstrated that one-third of patients did not receive the recommended immunizations, one-third did not receive the standard medicines for heart disease, and one-half did not receive the recommended care for diabetes.[40] Finally, *USA Today* printed an article entitled 'Doctors' care often deficient, study says' on the cover page on Thursday, June 26, 2003. This article emphasize three findings that support the article's title: patients with high blood pressure received 65% of recommended care, only 45% of heart attack patients received beta-blockers, and only a third of eligible patients had been screened for colorectal cancer.[41] Finally, a recent study by the American College of Chest Physicians showed that most family physicians and general internists are unfamiliar with the National Asthma Education and Prevention Program guidelines.[42]

Case 6.12 Protocols can be your saving grace

We believe that protocols were designed for a purpose and when a physician strays away from a protocol, she takes the associated risks that are described above. We had a patient who convinced us that protocols were designed for a purpose. A 69-year-old male came to the emergency department complaining of upper right chest pain after he had fallen off his motorcycle onto his right chest and shoulder. He had numerous coronary artery disease risk factors.

On initial presentation, he had reproducible pain in the involved areas and his right scapula, but there was no pain in his jaw or arms. There was also no diaphoresis, nausea, or vomiting. We ordered X-rays and an EKG. His nurse immediately gave us an inquisitive stare when she saw the EKG order. We told her of the protocol in Tintinalli's *Emergency Medicine: a comprehensive study guide.*[43] This protocol recommended an EKG within 10 minutes of arrival for all adult patients with chest pain. She was not able to perform the EKG immediately because the patient was taken to X-ray. Thirty minutes later, the patient returned with sweating and vomiting and an immediate EKG showed three millimeters of ST segment elevation in the anterior precordial lesions. The patient was taken immediately to the catheterization laboratory where he had angioplasty of his left anterior descending artery. Incidentally, he also had two broken ribs and a broken scapula on the right.

> ## Case 6.13 Tough to argue against protocols
>
> Pennachio writes in *Medical Economics* about a physician who used protocols to defend himself in a lawsuit.[44] A neurosurgeon was sued by a patient after complications from a carotid endarterectomy left her with permanent disability. The plaintiff claimed that the neurosurgeon did not discuss with her the option of chelation (EDTA) therapy in getting her informed consent for the procedure. The surgeon, however, showed that literature published by the American Medical Association, the American Heart Association, the American Academy of Family Physicians, the American College of Cardiology, and the American College of Physicians had opposed EDTA therapy in this context.[45] The verdict was in favor of the physician.

References

1 Horn C, Caldwell DH and Osborn DC (2000) *Law For Physicians: an overview of medical legal issues.* American Medical Association, Chicago, Illinois, 35–6.
2 Horn C, Caldwell DH and Osborn DC (2000) *Law For Physicians: an overview of medical legal issues.* American Medical Association, Chicago, Illinois, 36.
3 (1976) *The American Heritage Dictionary of the English Language, New College Edition.* Houghton Mifflin Company, Boston, Massachusetts, 378.
4 Horn C, Caldwell DH and Osborn DC (2000) *Law For Physicians: an overview of medical legal issues.* American Medical Association, Chicago, Illinois, 33.
5 Edwards FJ (2002) *The M & M Files: morbidity and mortality rounds in emergency medicine.* Hanley & Belfus Inc., Philadelphia, Pennsylvania, 190–92.
6 Edwards FJ (2002) *The M & M Files: morbidity and mortality rounds in emergency medicine.* Hanley & Belfus Inc., Philadelphia, Pennsylvania, 191–2.
7 Cohen H, Robinson ES and Mandrack M (2003) Getting to the root of medication errors: survey results. *Nursing 2003.* **33**(9): 36–45.
8 Cohen H, Robinson ES and Mandrack M (2003) Getting to the root of medication errors: survey results. *Nursing 2003.* **33**(9): 36.
9 Cohen H, Robinson ES and Mandrack M (2003) Getting to the root of medication errors: survey results. *Nursing 2003.* **33**(9): 38.
10 Cohen H, Robinson ES and Mandrack M (2003) Getting to the root of medication errors: survey results. *Nursing 2003.* **33**(9): 41.
11 Cohen H, Robinson ES and Mandrack M (2003) Getting to the root of medication errors: survey results. *Nursing 2003.* **33**(9): 41.
12 Cohen H, Robinson ES and Mandrack M (2003) Getting to the root of medication errors: survey results. *Nursing 2003.* **33**(9): 42.
13 Selbst SM and Korin JB (1999) *Preventing Malpractice Lawsuits in Pediatric Emergency Medicine.* American College of Emergency Physicians, Dallas, Texas, 87.
14 Doherty K, Segal A and McKinney PG (2004) The 10 most common prescribing errors: tips on avoiding the pitfalls. *Consultant.* **44**(2): 173–82.
15 Doherty K, Segal A and McKinney PG (2004) The 10 most common prescribing errors: tips on avoiding the pitfalls. *Consultant.* **44**(2): 173–4.
16 Doherty K, Segal A and McKinney PG (2004) The 10 most common prescribing errors: tips on avoiding the pitfalls. *Consultant.* **44**(2): 174.
17 Doherty K, Segal A and McKinney PG (2004) The 10 most common prescribing errors: tips on avoiding the pitfalls. *Consultant.* **44**(2): 174.
18 Doherty K, Segal A and McKinney PG (2004) The 10 most common prescribing errors: tips on avoiding the pitfalls. *Consultant.* **44**(2): 174–8.

19 Doherty K, Segal A and McKinney PG (2004) The 10 most common prescribing errors: tips on avoiding the pitfalls. *Consultant*. **44**(2): 178–81.

20 Pearlman MD and Tintinalli JE (1998) *Emergency Care of the Woman*. McGraw-Hill, New York, New York, 52.

21 Selbst SM and Korin JB (1999) *Preventing Malpractice Lawsuits in Pediatric Emergency Medicine*. American College of Emergency Physicians, Dallas, Texas, 122.

22 Edwards FJ (2002) *The M & M Files: morbidity and mortality rounds in emergency medicine*. Hanley & Belfus Inc., Philadelphia, Pennsylvania, 69–71.

23 Edwards FJ (2002) *The M & M Files: morbidity and mortality rounds in emergency medicine*. Hanley & Belfus Inc., Philadelphia, Pennsylvania, 71.

24 Edwards FJ (2002) *The M & M Files: morbidity and mortality rounds in emergency medicine*. Hanley & Belfus Inc., Philadelphia, Pennsylvania, 83–4.

25 Edwards FJ (2002) *The M & M Files: morbidity and mortality rounds in emergency medicine*. Hanley & Belfus Inc., Philadelphia, Pennsylvania, 83.

26 Edwards FJ (2002) *The M & M Files: morbidity and mortality rounds in emergency medicine*. Hanley & Belfus Inc., Philadelphia, Pennsylvania, 85–7.

27 Edwards FJ (2002) *The M & M Files: morbidity and mortality rounds in emergency medicine*. Hanley & Belfus Inc., Philadelphia, Pennsylvania, 86 .

28 Zobel HB and Rous SN (1993) *Doctors and the Law: defendants and expert witnesses* W Norton & Company, New York, New York.

29 Selbst SM and Korin JB (1999) *Preventing Malpractice Lawsuits in Pediatric Emergency Medicine*. American College of Emergency Physicians, Dallas, Texas.

30 Horn C, Caldwell DH and Osborn DC (2000) *Law For Physicians: an overview of medical legal issues*. American Medical Association, Chicago, Illinois.

31 Edwards FJ (2002) *The M & M Files: morbidity and mortality rounds in emergency medicine*. Hanley & Belfus Inc., Philadelphia, Pennsylvania.

32 Merry A and McCall Smith A (2001) *Errors, Medicine and the Law*. Cambridge University Press, Cambridge, United Kingdom.

33 Montague A (1996) *Legal Problems in Emergency Medicine*. Oxford University Press, Oxford, United Kingdom.

34 Edwards FJ (1989) *Medical Malpractice: solving the crisis*. Henry Holt and Company, New York, New York.

35 Rice B (2003) Are you liable for a colleague's mistake? *Medical Economics*. **80**(12): 33–42.

36 Horn C, Caldwell DH and Osborn DC (2000) *Law For Physicians: an overview of medical legal issues*. American Medical Association, Chicago, Illinois, 42.

37 Horn C, Caldwell DH and Osborn DC (2000) *Law For Physicians: an overview of medical legal issues*. American Medical Association, Chicago, Illinois, 43.

38 Nass C and Blumenthal RS (2003) Lipid management with HMG CoA reductase inhibitors in the elderly. *Annals of Long-Term Care*. **11**(6): 23.

39 Blomkalns AL (2003) *Modern Advances in Emergency Cardiac Care: evolution of diagnostic and treatment options*. EMCREG International, Cincinnati, Ohio, 30.

40 (2003) Doctors not following treatment guidelines: study. *Physicians Financial News*. **21**(10): 17.

41 Rubin R (2003) Doctors' care often deficient, study says. *USA Today*. **June 26**, 1A.

42 Peck P (2003) Half of primary care doctors don't follow asthma guidelines. *Family Practice News*. **33**(23): 22.

43 Tintinalli JE, Kelen GD and Stapczynski JS (2000) *Emergency Medicine: a comprehensive study guide* (5e). McGraw-Hill, New York, New York, 343.

44 Pennachio DL (2004) Clinical guidelines: sword or shield? *Medical Economics*. **81**(12): 22–3.

45 Pennachio DL (2004) Clinical guidelines: sword or shield? *Medical Economics*. **81**(12): 23.

Chapter 7

Clinical tips to decrease liability in your practice: part 2

- Follow hospital protocols
- Do not place over-reliance on test results
- Be receptive to assistance with pharmaceuticals
- Always review the prior chart for a 'bounce-back' patient
- Obtain old charts frequently
- Anticipate problems
- Review all stat labs before discharging a patient
- Know when and when not to let your patients play physician
- Be alert for commonly overlooked diagnoses
- Be punctual
- Dealing with the sympathy factor
- Instruct your staff on how to handle phone calls
- Listen carefully to questions from your triage nurse
- Do not leave medicine unattended and unsupervised
- There are times when textbooks are inaccurate or one reference may not be enough
- Be careful with patients on Coumadin
- Make sure that all of your medical staff introduce themselves to patients
- Chronic problems often require expedient work-ups

Follow hospital protocols

Most hospitals develop protocols for managing certain medical conditions. These protocols may vary from hospital to hospital. Although hospitals generally do not make it mandatory that their physicians follow their protocols strictly, it is usually advisable for physicians to adhere to them. Protocols are developed by committees composed of local physicians and are generally regarded as 'standard of care.' Therefore, therapies that are aberrant from written hospital protocols are difficult to defend in court. Furthermore, you can be assured that the plaintiff attorney will have a giant-sized poster of the protocol to show the court.

Case 7.1 Playing by house rules

Leinen and Guldner discuss a case, in *EMpulse*, where a physician could have lost a case if he had not followed hospital protocol.[1] This case involves the proper service to admit trauma patients. Some hospitals, including ours, have a protocol where all trauma patients are directed to the general or trauma surgery's service. The physician in this case, however, was fortunate that his hospital did not have such a protocol.

The patient is a 55-year-old man who fell six feet off a truck and struck his head, chest, and left arm on the ground. He was not certain whether he lost consciousness and complained of chest pain, headache, and low back pain. The ED physician noted that he had mild trouble breathing because of the chest pain. His vitals on presentation were unremarkable except for mild tachypnea with a respiratory rate of 24 breaths/minute.

Significant findings on physical exam included a 9 cm laceration in the left parietal scalp area and extreme tenderness over the left mid thoracic ribs. His neurologic examination was unremarkable. The chest X-ray showed fractured ribs on the left but no pneumothorax. The head CT scan showed a small subdural hematoma and a non-displaced skull fracture. The patient's blood work was unremarkable. He was then admitted to the neurosurgical service with the diagnoses of: blunt head and chest trauma, multiple rib fractures, non-depressed skull fracture, subdural hematoma, and a cerebral contusion.

The patient's hospital course grew increasingly complicated. He was treated with intravenous narcotics, which contributed to the development of an ileus. The ileus along with its accompanying abdominal distention, in combination with respiratory splinting from the rib fractures, led to severe respiratory difficulties. A trauma consult was obtained at this time and the patient was then intubated and placed on a mechanical ventilator. He continued to require the use of a mechanical ventilator for almost two weeks. This prolonged course led to the development of subglottal stenosis and the inability to return to his usual job or engage in any strenuous activity.

The patient subsequently filed a lawsuit against the emergency physician. The plaintiff attorney's argument was that his patient should have been admitted to the trauma service. It was also implied that the patient's complications from multi-system trauma might not have occurred if the trauma team had been involved early in the course of hospitalization. Specifically, they felt that the patient should have received a nasogastric tube to relieve his abdominal distention and he should have received better pain management for his rib fractures.

The defense, however, argued that the patient had mainly a neurosurgical problem on admission and was admitted to the appropriate service. They stated that the emergency physician was board-certified and qualified to determine the appropriate service to admit the patient. He also felt that the patient did not need a trauma consult on admission. Furthermore, they felt that the trauma team would have likely signed the patient off to the neurosurgery team based on the admitting diagnoses.

continued

The verdict in this case was in favor of the defense. This case is a good example of an increasing trend in malpractice cases. The majority of malpractice cases have traditionally been for misdiagnosis, complications from procedures, and medication complications. Lawsuits are increasingly filed, however, for errors in treatment decisions such as the case filed above. The contention of the plaintiff attorney in the above case was that the ED physician fell below the standard of care by not admitting the patient to the trauma service.

Therefore, it is extremely important to follow hospital or departmental protocols. They serve as an equivalent to the standard of care. Leinen and Guidner write, in *EMpulse*, 'if a policy exists that specifies when exactly a trauma consult should be obtained, then the EP could be in trouble. Very often hospitals develop policies that may not be known to all of the staff. If a policy was in place that required the emergency physician to obtain a consult, he may have well lost the case.'[2]

Do not place over-reliance on test results

Diagnostic tests were designed to assist the physician with evaluating the patient's illness. We would all probably agree that we would much rather practice medicine today with our high technology equipment, than practice 100 years ago when physicians had to rely more on their clinical skills and intuition. However, tests and labs can be double-edged swords if one is not aware of their limitations, their indications, their accuracy, or their precision.

There is no perfect test in medicine. This is because tests are designed by people, for people, and interpreted by people. Therefore they are subject to the same limitations that people are. You should have a rough estimate of the sensitivity and specificity of the tests that you order. In addition, you should be aware of conditions that will produce a false positive (e.g. congestive heart failure producing a positive ventilation/perfusion lung scan) or a false negative (e.g. gallbladder ultrasound performed after a patient has eaten a full meal).

Furthermore, there are many conditions where diagnostic tests are frequently normal despite the presence of serious medical emergencies. In these circumstances, acceptance of test results without consideration of the clinical context of the patient can result in extremely high liability situations. More specifically, the scenarios that we have seen physicians 'get burned' on the most due to overdependence on test results are acute abdominal pain, acute stroke symptoms, and acute chest pain. Acute infections in the abdomen requiring surgical intervention frequently are associated with an elevated white blood cell count or abnormal imaging. However, when the infection is in the early stages or is in an atypical location, both of these tests will have reduced sensitivity.

Symptoms of acute stroke or transient ischemic attacks are frequently evaluated with a CT scan of the head. However, experience has taught us that the majority of these patients will have a negative CT scan on initial presentation. The low sensitivity of this test can be falsely reassuring to the inexperienced physician.

Case 7.2 But the test was negative

A new ED physician recently sent a patient with left-sided numbness home after the CT scan of the head was negative. Although the patient had objective findings of weakness and was concerned about having a stroke, the doctor informed him that it was not possible because his head CT was normal. The patient returned the next day with symptoms of a progressive stroke with left-sided weakness and ischemic changes on the second CT scan of the head.

The last example is a common one for emergency physicians. This is the patient who presents with symptoms suggestive of cardiac ischemia, or has cardiac risk factors. The emergency evaluation of these patients will frequently reveal a normal EKG and normal cardiac enzymes. These findings, however, must not override the suspicion of cardiac ischemia if the presentation is worrisome or if there is a significant amount of cardiac risk factors. We believe that almost every emergency physician can personally relay a case of a 'missed MI (myocardial infarction)' due to over-reliance on tests.

Be receptive to assistance with pharmaceuticals

Similar to the comments in the above section, medications were designed to make patients better. However, when incorrectly or mistakenly given, they can produce grave medical and legal consequences. Lawsuits concerning drug administration represent a significant portion of medical malpractice cases. Furthermore, these types of suits are more difficult to defend because they usually represent an objective error by the healthcare provider(s) and that is portrayed as unacceptable to the judge and jury.

With this in mind, we must utilize every available avenue to prevent drug errors (although those of us that have practiced for a significant amount of time know that one cannot eliminate them completely and they will sometimes happen). Fortunately for us, there are many back-up mechanisms in the health system to assist in avoiding medication errors. Nurses and pharmacists both review medication orders. In addition, sometimes computers or other physicians will also review medication orders. An overt error in the wording of an order or a script is frequently picked up by one of these ancillary medical personnel. In addition, pharmacists will often remind you of a drug interaction or nurses will remind you that the patient is allergic to the medication. When these medical colleagues come to your assistance, be receptive and attentive to their concerns even if you are already aware of it. By doing so, you will encourage them to help you in the future when they just may be able to save you from a lawsuit or from losing your license. In contrast, a condescending, inattentive attitude may leave you without a back-up system in the future.

Always review the prior chart for a 'bounce-back' patient

With the exception of the simplest cases, it is usually beneficial to obtain previous charts in patients who return for repeat evaluations for the same complaints. For example, if a patient returns stating no improvement because she did not get her medications filled, she will probably not require an extensive evaluation or review of prior testing. However, most will return because they have had a change in their condition or they were misdiagnosed. Therefore it will be helpful to review their prior evaluations for several purposes.

Earlier in this chapter, we talked about 'two heads being better than one.' Skimming through a prior chart to get a feel of what the prior physician was thinking will give you another perspective of the patient's problems. This second opinion will assist you in formulating a broader approach to your evaluation unless you automatically assume that the prior physician was correct or incorrect. In addition, knowledge of the prior tests that were performed helps you decide which ones to repeat, which ones not to repeat, which ones to add, and which ones to use in comparison. Finally, since the patient is not better, it will be important to see if she followed the discharge instructions and took the prescribed medications given by the prior physician.

There will be times when obtaining the old chart is not possible. The chart may have been sent to the coders for billing. The prior evaluation may have taken place at another facility, etc. Although the treating physician may be aware of the unlikely possibility of obtaining the record, she should still write an order for it on the chart and have the staff make at least one honest attempt. The order for old records or other evidence of data request such as consent for release of medical records may be your saving grace in court if an adverse outcome occurs as a result of your not having knowledge from a prior visit.

Case 7.3 When things are not better

Edwards presents a case, in *The M & M Files*, where a review of the prior chart would have been helpful during a repeat evaluation.[3] This case also is relevant to the prior section regarding a step-up in care in return patients. A 19-year-old lady presented to the ED with painful urination for two days. She did not have any other associated symptoms. She appeared in no distress and had no abdominal or flank tenderness on examination. The clean catch urine result showed greater than 25 white blood cells, a few red blood cells and epithelial cells. A pregnancy test done on the urine was negative. She was discharged with sulfamethoxazole-trimethoprim and pyridium for a urinary tract infection (UTI).

The patient's symptoms worsened and she returned to the ED the following day. The second ED physician looked in the computer to see if the urine culture results were available and found that it was not ordered. He assumed that the patient's 'UTI' was due to a resistant organism and changed the antibiotic to ciprofloxacin. He also left a note to the first ED physician questioning why a urine culture was not ordered.

The symptoms were even worse the next day when the patient once again

continued

returned to the ED. The third ED physician took a more extensive history and found it strange that the patient had no associated symptoms of a UTI such as urinary urgency or frequency. Instead, the patient told him that the burning was more present when the urine hit the outside. Upon hearing this, the physician performed a pelvic exam and discovered that the patient had findings consistent with herpes genitalis. He discovered vesicles, ulceration, and swelling around the labia and introitus.

Urinary tract infections in sexually active females are extremely common and most patients who present for them do not want or expect to have a pelvic exam. It is always helpful to ask the patient if she has a history of UTIs or whether the current symptoms are similar to her prior UTIs. If the answer to either question is no, a pelvic examination should probably be recommended. In addition, any suggestion of a genital-related etiology such as vaginal discharge, vaginal swelling, and vaginal lesions warrants a pelvic examination.

We believe that the first ED physician probably gave an appropriate evaluation for this patient. He might have performed a more complete evaluation by taking a more extensive history and not regarding this patient as a 30-second 'treat and street' patient. The second physician, however, did not render an appropriate evaluation. He did not take the time to review the old chart and develop a broader approach to the evaluation. He focused on why the 'UTI' was not better and did not obtain a better history or perform a step-up in examination with a pelvic exam (which would have been indicated in a bounce-back patient). He also considered himself an authority on management of UTIs by criticizing the first physician for not ordering a urine culture. This practice is well published in the current medical literature as not being cost-effective for the routine evaluation for UTIs.

Obtain old charts frequently

This is an extension of the concept of the previous section. It would be ideal to treat every patient with her medical chart available for review. This is impossible, however, due to the limitations of the physician and the limitations of the practice. Physicians do not have the time to review every patient's chart in the average 15 minutes that is allotted for each patient. Furthermore, not every patient or every patient visit requires a review of the patient's medical history. For example, some patients are well prepared for their physician encounter and can provide (either verbally or in writing) every medical detail that you ask. Visits such as for those for lacerations or prescription refills generally do not require that the physician be familiar with the patient's prior medical history.

As we discussed in the prior section, every medical practice has exceptions where an old chart cannot be accessed. Even in practices where we have worked like the Veterans Administration Hospital when all medical documentation is entered into the computer, there are considerable periods in which the computer system is down for reprogramming, and accessing medical records, thus, becomes impossible. We have also discussed in earlier chapters some alternative sources for obtaining prior medical records.

For what types of patients do we usually request medical records? Patients who have multiple chronic medical problems and who are on multiple medications represent the majority of this group. We may need to know the latest interventions for their chronic medical problems (e.g. percutaneous coronary intervention for coronary artery disease). We may look for medications that they are taking which may require us to check levels. Finally, we may look for other medical complications that could arise from their chronic medical conditions. The last group of patients for whom we typically request old charts include: patients who are unable to give a history, patients who may give false histories, psychiatric and non-compliant patients, and patients recently discharged from the hospital (to look for complications from medical treatment of their recent condition).

Case 7.4 Finding treasures in the chart

The following case illustrates the benefit of reviewing an old chart. A 65-year-old woman with a history of congestive heart failure (CHF) presented to the ED complaining of an exacerbation of her CHF. She noted that her legs had developed increased swelling and that she had gotten progressively more short of breath in the past week. She was on a long list of medications but did not know their names; instead, she told the ED physician to get her chart because she had been to our hospital numerous times. The ED physician did not feel that this was necessary because he felt that he could treat this woman's symptoms and probably discharge her.

Indeed, the ED physician ordered some screening cardiac tests and gave the woman intravenous diuretics and subsequently discharged her home. She returned to the ED two nights later and was seen by us. She had the same complaints and the same presentation and requested to be admitted to the hospital. We requested her old chart to discover more information about her (i.e. her medications, her compliance record, her other medical problems). We discovered that she was also taking Coumadin for chronic atrial fibrillation and digoxin for her congestive heart failure. In addition, we discovered that her previous hospitalization approximately one year ago was for a rapidly expanding abdominal aortic aneurysm (AAA). It was almost 6 cm in diameter at the time but she was evaluated by vascular surgery as a poor candidate for surgical repair. We ordered the same tests and same medications as the first physician with the additions of a digoxin level and an International Normalized Ratio (INR). The digoxin level was almost undetectable and the INR was 7.

Although our evaluation showed that the patient probably did not need to be admitted for her congestive heart failure because it was well compensated, she did require admission for her other medical problems. In her case, an AAA of this size is at high risk for rupture and rapid exsanguinations with her coagulopathy. Therefore, she was admitted to the hospital to have this coagulopathy corrected. This medical problem was not one for which the patient presented to the ED but was one that was discovered by review of the patient's chart (a task that the patient had requested on the first visit).

Anticipate problems

The practice of medicine is not only about treating problems but it also involves the anticipation of potential problems. Medical conditions that arise at a later time but have a foundation based on prior visits have become increasing sources of litigation in recent years. Common examples that we have included elsewhere in this book include protecting the suicidal patient from killing herself, preventing the patient who has been given intravenous narcotics from driving, and not permitting a head injury patient who lives alone to go home unsupervised. Prudent anticipation of medical problems was a skill that could only be acquired through experience in the past. With the increased interest in case-based medical publications (such as this text), however, it is now easier for physicians to learn about potential difficulties without having the first-hand experience.

Case 7.5 I should have seen it coming

Edwards presents a case, in *The M & M Files*, where anticipation by the physician would have avoided a complaint.[4] A 47-year-old woman with a long history of severe asthma requiring numerous hospitalizations presented to the ED with three days of vomiting and diarrhea. She had been on steroids chronically for the past six months for her asthma but was otherwise healthy. She presented with a tired appearance, dry oral mucous membranes, and was tachycardic with a rate of 115 beats/minute. The rest of her vital signs, however, were normal and her abdominal exam was benign.

During her stay in the ED, she received intravenous fluids and nausea medicine. A complete blood count and complete metabolic panel were sent and were both normal with the exception of a mildly elevated blood urea nitrogen. The nausea improved, the diarrhea stopped, and she was able to tolerate fluids in the ED. At this time, she was discharged with the diagnosis of 'nonspecific gastroenteritis' and given a prescription for Tigan suppositories and told to use Pepto-Bismol if the diarrhea returned. No other instructions were given.

During the next two days, the patient was unable to hold anything down (including her medications) and she became lethargic and weak. Her husband decided to take her to a different ED because he was frustrated with the first ED for discharging her. The patient was admitted at the second hospital for dehydration and adrenal crisis secondary to steroid withdrawal. Although she did well with intravenous fluids and steroids, her husband filed a complaint against the first ED physician (on the recommendation of the second ED physician) for not addressing the potential problem of vomiting while taking steroids chronically.

Although we cannot find fault with anything that the first ED physician did during his medical treatment of this patient, his error came in his failure to anticipate a potential problem in this patient on chronic steroids. Despite the frustration of the patient's husband at her discharge, the release was probably appropriate since her symptoms had improved and she was able

continued

to hold down oral intake in the ED. We believe that the complaint would probably have been avoided if the first ED physician had stressed to the patient the importance of her taking the steroids and to return immediately if any vomiting returned.

Review all stat labs before discharging a patient

This statement may sound very simple, but it is sometimes not easy to follow. Some patients may become frustrated while waiting for labs and may request to leave. Other patients feel better after a therapeutic intervention and would like to go home. They may also try to persuade you to call them with the lab results. Physicians are often encouraged to release patients prematurely so that other patients may be seen. Finally, physicians sometimes lose track of the labs that they order. This last event is not uncommon in a busy emergency department where a physician may have over 100 labs pending at one time.

There are many potential problems with discharging a patient before all of the stat labs are returned. The most obvious one is the abnormal lab that needs to be addressed immediately. Some patients may not leave a contact number or address, while others may live hours away and cannot be contacted on the road. We have experienced that even when we are able to contact patients, a good number of them do not have transportation to return. Do not forget the additional time of finding the chart and making the phone call. Finally, the patient may be left with the impression that her physician is incompetent.

The second reason is that although some labs may not require immediate attention, the patient should be aware of the result. The most common example of this is the female who comes with urinary symptoms or upper abdominal pain and is found to have a positive pregnancy test after discharge. Although it is highly doubtful, in these situations, that the pregnancy has anything to do with the patient's symptoms, there are large implications for the patient's lack of awareness of her pregnancy. She may take medications that are contraindicated in pregnancy or drink excessive alcohol. Her prenatal care may be delayed. Finally, in the unfortunate scenario, she may have an ectopic pregnancy that may rupture and lead to death.

The last reason to hold patients until all stat labs are received is for legal purposes. The legal community generally views the discharge of patients with uncertainty of their labs as substandard practice. Furthermore, hospital review committees and insurance company reviewers may question why labs are ordered stat if they are not going to affect the disposition.

Case 7.6 Unfinished business

Edwards presents a case, in *The M & M Files*, where the premature discharge of a patient led to a physician's reprimand.[5] A 63-year-old woman presented to the ED with the complaints of weakness, dizziness, nausea, anorexia, and intermittent fevers. Despite a temperature of 100.9°F and a

continued

pulse of 116 beats/minute, the rest of her physical exam was unremarkable. The patient's complete blood count and her basic serum chemistries were normal. The complete metabolic panel was still pending when the patient was feeling better after a dose of meclizine and oral fluids. The patient was discharged with the diagnosis of 'viral syndrome with labyrinthitis' and given a prescription for meclizine.

Shortly after the patient left, the rest of her labs returned. The ED physician was surprised to find that her total bilirubin was 4.1 mg/dl and her liver enzymes were elevated. The physician made an attempt to contact the patient but was unsuccessful. He discovered later that the patient had fainted after she had returned home and that her husband had taken her to a different ED. He became aware of these events when he received a complaint from the patient's husband.

Many of the issues that we discussed above are relevant to this case. The ED physician stated that he was under pressure from the nurses to release the patient. The callback attempt was unsuccessful. A possible reason might have been that the patient was being taken to another hospital at the time. Finally, the patient and her husband are not satisfied with the early release and probably are left believing that the physician is incompetent.

Case 7.7 Clearing them out too quickly

We endured an embarrassing experience in our emergency department when we did not follow this rule. A 48-year-old male bodybuilder came to our ED after having an hour episode of severe chest pain that had resolved 15 minutes prior to his presentation. He wrote chest pain on his triage note and told the triage nurse that it felt like 'someone sitting on [his] chest.' He pointed, however, to the epigastric area when we saw him. The pain did not radiate to his jaw or arms. There was sweating but no nausea or vomiting. His past medical history and family history were negative for coronary artery disease risk factors. He had a 20-year history of tobacco use but recently quit. The physical examination was completely unremarkable.

In the ED, his EKG had QS complexes in leads III and AVF and poor R wave progression in the precordial leads. Complete blood count, cardiac enzymes, and chest X-ray were all unremarkable. We also ordered amylase and lipase because of his localization of the pain to the epigastrium. The patient had no further pain, no EKG changes, and we contacted the cardiologist on call. After reviewing the EKGs by fax, the cardiologist decided to admit the patient. We had already stayed one hour over our shift to finish up on some patients, so we were excited to leave once the patient was admitted.

When we returned to the hospital the following day, we found out that the patient's lipase was 850 international units/liter and he had acute pancreatitis. We had forgotten to check on this lab once he was admitted to the hospital. We were also told that the ED physician on duty during the night wanted to admit him for pancreatitis but that he had signed out against medical advice because he had no medical insurance. We were saved the embarrassment because the cardiologist was not notified of this diagnosis.

Know when and when not to let your patients play physician

Due to the popularity and increased availability of the internet, patients have a great deal of access to medical information. Many will come to your office with preconceptions of their medical diagnoses. They will often express these opinions and try to influence you with them. While some of these opinions may be correct and helpful, others may be inaccurate and distracting to the correct diagnoses. The astute physician must decipher which opinions to accept and which to reject.

Patients with chronic or recurrent medical problems are usually familiar with the presenting symptoms of their illnesses. Hence they are often correct and their input is usually helpful. A typical example would be the patient with a prior myocardial infarction who presents with the same symptoms and believes she is having another myocardial infarction. She is probably right. Similarly, a patient that has a history of kidney stones who presents with the same type of symptoms as a prior attack can probably guess her diagnosis correctly. When the patients above present with symptoms that they state are not like their prior events, however, they should, likewise, be taken seriously and alternative diagnoses should be entertained.

In contrast to the situations above, patients who are presenting with symptoms suggestive of a new diagnosis are not uncommonly incorrect. The treating physician should not let the patient's preconceived diagnoses narrow her thought process. We have seen this happen so many times with inexperienced physicians. The classic example is the patient with risk factors for coronary artery disease (but no established diagnosis) who presents with chest pain and states that she feels that it is due to 'gas.' She may add that it is worse after she eats or that it is better with antacids. The physician may be lured into these suggestions and be distracted from the patient's coronary artery disease risk factors. Remember that in any profession, inexperience must be accepted with extreme caution. This also applies to the profession of being a patient.

Case 7.8 Should I listen to this patient?

An example from our experiences concerns a 23-year-old female who came into our emergency department with the acute onset of abdominal pain with vomiting and diarrhea. She presented with 24 hours of periumbilical pain and multiple bouts of vomiting and diarrhea without blood. She did not have any fevers but was tachycardic and hypotensive on initial exam. There was no prior history of gastrointestinal problems or abdominal surgeries. She stated: 'I know what the problem is; this all started after I ate some crabs yesterday.' She felt that she did not need any diagnostic tests and just needed some intravenous fluids.

She did not appear in significant distress on her physical exam and her abdomen had mild tenderness in the periumbilical area without guarding or rebound. A rectal exam did not reveal any blood in the stool. Routine blood work was sent and revealed a white blood cell count of 29 600

continued

cells/microliter with a normal differential. The rest of the blood work was unremarkable. A plain film of the abdomen did not reveal any free air or gas pattern suggestive of bowel obstruction. A CT scan of the abdomen, however, revealed inflammation and bowel wall thickening of her ileum with ulcerations. She was admitted to the gastroenterology service where subsequent bowel biopsies from colonoscopy were consistent with the diagnosis of Crohn's disease.

It is important to comment that individuals in the medical profession are often the biggest culprits. Nurses, medical assistants, paramedics, and other healthcare employees often visit you with their diagnosis already established in their mind. Some will not welcome a diagnostic evaluation and are only seeking treatment for their preconceived problem. They can sound extremely convincing and can, thus, cause you to deviate from your normal protocol.

Case 7.9 A patient's misdiagnosis

A second example is found in Edwards' *The M & M Files*.[6] A 60-year-old came to the ED after doing some farm work complaining of swelling, redness, and itching of the right side of his face. He had induration of his right cheek and swelling of his right periorbital area. He was not febrile and the area was not warm to touch. There were also some blisters on his right cheek and nose. Although the ED physician was unsure of the diagnosis, he agreed when the patient suggested that it might be poison ivy. Therefore, he sent the patient home with a tapered course of steroids.

The patient developed more blisters and more pain in his right eye over the next two days. He went to see his primary physician who diagnosed him with shingles and referred him to an ophthalmologist. Here, he was given the additional diagnosis of zoster ophthalmicus. The primary physician told the patient that the misdiagnosis should not have been made and this led to the patient filing a complaint to the hospital board against the ED physician.

The most important learning issue from this case is to not let your patient's impression of his medical condition obscure your medical reasoning. This case would have been extremely atypical for poison ivy. Poison ivy more commonly starts on the extremities and does not commonly involve only one side of the face. Furthermore, the clinical description of the lesions is not usual for poison ivy. Vesicles, when found on clinical exam, should immediately cause concern for herpetic infection. Remember that when the diagnosis is incorrect, it is the physician who made a poor judgment and not the patient.

We would like to add that the primary physician should consider whether his criticism is fair. He was able to see the patient after the outbreak was much more obvious and the diagnosis was much easier to make. This is how many lawsuits concerning medical malpractice initiate. Would the

continued

primary physician like it if another physician had questioned his judgment every time he had missed a diagnosis? In fact, Edwards points out that 'the first case of medical malpractice on record in English common law was generated when a second physician disparaged the care given by another physician for a hand injury (Stratton vs. Swanlond, 1375).'[7]

Case 7.10 Too early to tell

We had a personal experience similar to the preceding case. One morning, our mother called us to tell us that she had a severe headache on the left side of her face for two days. With her history of diabetes and hypertension, we became concerned of a serious etiology to her headache. Her pain did not improve over the next 24 hours. She noticed, however, a small papule that developed on the left side of her face. She had been gardening the previous few days and believed that an insect bite was causing her pain. Although we were relieved to hear this, we told her to go to the emergency department for a CT scan (for intracranial hemorrhage) of the head and a sedimentation rate (for temporal arteritis).

The emergency physician on duty was extremely amicable when we told him that she was coming in. He ordered the tests that we wanted and examined her. Her physical exam did not reveal any other significant finding except the papule. The results of her tests were all normal. He discussed with us his plans for starting her on antibiotics for the insect bite. Everyone was relieved and satisfied.

Two days later, she continued to have the severe pain. We told her to go to her family physician for a recheck. Her family physician made the diagnosis immediately upon looking at her. She now had three vesicles on the left side of her face in a dermatomal distribution. The cause was a herpes zoster eruption. She was treated without complications. Her family physician was an extremely proud man because he made a diagnosis immediately without the assistance of expensive tests. He took photographs for his clinical files.

We certainly have much respect for her physician for his clinical acuity. However, he also benefited from seeing her after the diagnosis had became more obvious. In addition, we believe that emergency department tests were valid and justified in our mother's initial presentation. Although we cannot expect patients to always share this same viewpoint, we must be careful about criticizing other physicians (as in the above case) unjustifiably.

Be alert for commonly overlooked diagnoses

Certain diagnoses have the tendency to be overlooked for several reasons. They may present with several clinical manifestations without one predominating, which may decrease the physician's focus towards a specific diagnosis. The symptoms may develop in a gradual and progressive nature, making it difficult for the physician to track or associate the evolution. The diagnosis may not be definitely made by one specific test or requires a specific test that is not routinely available. In some instances, test results may not be immediately available.

Although the majority of these overlooked diagnoses do not represent emergencies, they can create medical liability when there are associated complications from prolonged misdiagnoses. A recent article in *Patient Care* journal also discussed this topic.[8] The authors described six conditions that are commonly overlooked in primary care. They also offer reasons why these conditions are often not diagnosed.

1 Malignant melanoma is often not suspected in younger patients. This is despite the fact that it is a more common cancer in the 25 to 29-year-old age group than any other non-skin cancer.
2 Aortic stenosis may be missed during its prolonged asymptomatic period despite significant stenosis.
3 Appendicitis may be confused with many other gastrointestinal and gynecological disease processes.
4 The early signs and symptoms of meningitis may be subtle and may not be the classic ones (stiff neck, vomiting) that we expect.
5 The evaluation of depression may be misdirected at the patient's accompanying somatic complaints.
6 Finally, the symptoms of thyroid dysfunction may be misleading because they typically start slowly.

Be punctual

Punctuality is important in almost any job, but especially in the medical profession. Patients in the office have appointment times, while physicians who do shift work must relieve their colleagues from their duties. Tardiness is not only likely to create frustration among others, but it can also be detrimental to one's responsibilities. We encountered an unfortunate case of this in our residency.

Case 7.11 Day late and dollar short

During our residency, we were able to moonlight as house officers for a hospital which was specialized for patients with respiratory disease who are on mechanical ventilators. Our role as house officers was to be on the hospital premises from 7 pm to 7 am and respond to any cardiac or pulmonary arrest that occurred on our shift. This event occurred very infrequently because most of the patients at the hospital had a 'do not resuscitate' order. The residents in our program had negotiated a contract with this hospital to provide coverage every day of the year.

One resident had a persistent habit of arriving late for his shift. His tardiness could range from 20 minutes to five hours. He just seemed to report to work whenever his social plans were completed. This behavior went unnoticed by the hospital for over one year because their records

---

continued

showed that his recorded hours were 7 pm to 7 am with all of his shifts. A few of us were aware of his antics and we repeatedly told him that he would 'get burned' eventually. We, however, did not report him because he was 'one of the boys.'

One night, a code blue (cardiac arrest) was called at 7:20 pm. Resuscitative efforts were attempted without success and without the presence of a licensed physician. The physician that was scheduled was our infamous resident who was not present until midnight. The event never instigated any hospital review. Our resident group, however, voted to take away some of this resident's shifts. Unfortunately, this punishment was not enough because the resident did not mend his tardy ways. The lesson of punctuality, however, was an extremely important one for the rest of us.

Dealing with the sympathy factor

Physicians who have been sued know how important the sympathy factor is. When a patient suffers a permanent injury or death, the defense of the physician becomes much more difficult in court because of the sympathy factor. Jurors may become emotionally biased when they see a disabled patient who is not able to care for herself. Likewise, when they see the widow and young kids of a deceased patient, they sympathize with how the family will survive. Plaintiff attorneys will do everything that they can to highlight the injury or disability to the jurors. They may bring the patient into the courtroom and parade her in front of the jurors. They may show videotapes of how the injuries have affected the patient's life.

Case 7.12 A picture is worth a thousand words

We once heard a story from another physician that he was being sued for not making the diagnosis of colon cancer in a timely fashion. His patient was now dying from colon cancer but the plaintiff attorney was delaying the trial. The defense's speculation was that the plaintiff attorney was waiting until the patient died so that he could make a more dramatic presentation in the courtroom with the widow and two young children.

Case 7.13 A difficult sight to watch

An excellent article on this subject was found in the *Medical Economics* journal.[9] The case example in this article was a $7.6 million judgment against a Florida obstetrician. The plaintiff was a seven-year-old boy with cerebral palsy whom the physician had delivered. Although there was significant controversy regarding the doctor's negligence in the case, the jury became sympathetic to the patient when he was brought into the courtroom and waved to the jurors. The large amount of the award was partly to cover the cost of his continuous care and metal leg braces for support.

Cases like this where there is a sympathy factor have frustrated defense attorneys and physicians for years. Some very prominent defense attorneys offer advice in this article on neutralizing the sympathy factor. The 'power points' from this article are:

1 Establish your credibility with the jury by recognizing the severity of the patient's injury.
2 Admit that what happened to the patient is devastating, and that jurors' feelings of sympathy are perfectly natural.
3 Don't get angry; showing anger makes you appear cold and uncaring.
4 Show the jury that you're a person as well as a physician.[10]

The article also discusses some techniques that defense attorneys have used to minimize the impact of a severely injured plaintiff. One attorney uses the direct approach by telling the jurors that they will become emotional and moved. He then reminds them that the judge has advised them to not let their emotions influence their decisions. Finally, he encourages them to make their decisions based solely on the facts.[10]

Another attorney claims that 'the way to deal with the emotional effect is not to fight, minimize, or ignore it.'[10] He feels it is best to give everyone in the court-room the permission to sympathize with the patient's injuries. He also stresses that his client shares the same sympathy as the others in the courtroom.

Some attorneys have found it helpful to request the presence of the injured plaintiff during jury selection. Their reasoning is that although most jurors will say that they can be impartial when the patient is not there, their feelings often change when they actually see the patient. Witnessing the jurors' response in the presence of the patient helps these attorneys make better jury selections.

The article also discusses techniques that can be used by physicians to counter the sympathy factor.[11] The most obvious one is to make your compassion for the patient readily apparent to everyone in the courtroom. The second one is for the physician to personalize herself. Let people know that you are also a wife with children or a daughter with a mother in the same manner as members of the jury. Give them the impression that you are a family person with the same morals and concerns. Finally, tell the jury how much time you spent with your patient and her family.

Instruct your staff on how to handle phone calls

Physician practices consist of a diverse group of employees. Secretaries, medical assistants, nurses, radiology technicians, electrocardiogram technicians, and respiratory technicians can all be constituents of this group. At a given point in time, any member of this group may answer the phone and listen to a patient's questions. The amount of training in phone triage is extremely varied among these staff members. Therefore, incorrect and damaging information may be given to patients inadvertently.

Physicians must instruct their staff on the types of information that they can and cannot give over the phone. If there is any doubt to a patient's question, the physician should always be openly available for consultation. It is also good practice to have a nurse well trained in phone triage field the majority of phone calls. In this way, experienced advice can be disseminated and proper documentation made.

Two examples of inappropriate information given over the phone are from our office.

Case 7.14 'Uncommon' sense advice

A young man who was diagnosed with sinusitis one week ago called and stated that he was still having the 'sinus headaches.' He wanted a refill of the antibiotics and the pain medicine that was prescribed previously. The secretary who answered the phone remembered that the office's policy in general was not to refill antibiotics over the phone. She therefore told the patient that his medications could not be refilled without him coming to the office for a recheck. The patient became upset and said that he was not going to come in for more antibiotics. He then asked the secretary what he should take for the sinus headaches. The secretary reflexively replied that he should take aspirin. The patient became more enraged and filed a complaint against the clinic because he was allergic to aspirin.

Case 7.15 A sensitive issue

The second concerns a patient that called the office requesting a prescription of Viagra. He had obtained some samples from a friend and now wanted his own prescription. He had not had an evaluation for sexual dysfunction at our office, however. We instructed the nurse to call the patient and have him come in to be seen. She, in turn, delegated this duty to the secretary. When the secretary called his home number, she told a female over a phone that the patient needed to be seen before he could get a script for Viagra. We discovered later from a complaint from the patient that the lady was his wife and that they were temporarily separated.

Listen carefully to questions from your triage nurse

This is a corollary statement to the previous statement. In the emergency department, it is equally important to have adequately trained staff to handle phone triage. The severity of the pathology and the lack of familiarity with the patient increase the likelihood of mistakes during phone triage. Patients will often call back when a different physician is working who is unaware of the events of the patient's visit. Therefore, it is critical for the triage nurse to obtain the necessary information from the visit and present it appropriately to the physician on duty. The physician, in turn, should carefully review a chart whenever a patient is not doing better or is doing worse. If there is no clear reason why the patient has not improved, she should be instructed to return for further evaluation.

Case 7.16 The warning call

Edwards presents a case, in *The M & M Files*, where a patient's phone call was not carefully reviewed.[12] After a pile of railroad ties fell off a forklift and pinned his legs, a 59-year-old man presented to the emergency department. The patient had pain and swelling in his legs but his neurovascular examination was normal. X-rays performed on the lower extremities were unremarkable. The patient was discharged with pain medicine and instructed to follow up with the occupational medicine clinic in three days.

The patient's pain grew worse later that night prompting his wife to call the ED for advice. After the triage nurse pulled his chart and spoke briefly with the physician on duty, she informed the wife that the radiologist had reviewed the films and did not see a fracture. She also recommended that the patient elevate his legs and increase his pain medicines.

The patient returned to the ED approximately 36 hours later with tense swelling in his legs and questionable distal pulses in his legs. He was immediately diagnosed with compartment syndrome and the orthopedist was called to see him. After confirmation by compartment pressure measurements, the patient was taken to the operating room. He was found to have significant muscle damage and required extensive debridement. The patient filed a lawsuit and received a large settlement from the hospital.

The physician on duty during the callback recalled only that the triage nurse asked him 'whether a patient with a contusion and increased pain could take two pills at once.'[13] It is easy to see how a physician may not give such a question deep thought. On the other hand, worsening pain should always be a red flag for a physician to investigate for the cause. The problem could have also been avoided had the treating physician anticipated this potential complication in her discharge instructions and informed the patient to return immediately if his pain worsens.

Do not leave medicine unattended and unsupervised

We all know that medicines can be harmful if taken inappropriately. In general, patients should be taking only medicines that are prescribed to them by a physician. This is not always the case, however, as there are many other ways in which patients can obtain medicine. In our practice, we have seen nurses and office staff remove medicines from the sample cabinet without talking to a physician. Patients are sometimes instructed to stop a medicine and will leave this medicine in the office without properly disposing of it. Lastly, pharmaceutical representatives frequently leave samples on countertops and physicians frequently leave medicine in the exam rooms.

A frequent example is that of ophthalmic analgesics. Complaints of eye pain are common and are usually medicated with analgesic eye drops. Ophthalmologist, however, generally recommend against the prescription of analgesic eye drops for home use for fear of masking a worsening condition. Patients, however, do not understand this and are only aware of the wonderful relief that they got in your office. Therefore, even after you tell them that you are not going to prescribe it to them and explain to them why, do not be surprised if a bottle of analgesic that is left unattended is suddenly gone when you return.

Case 7.17 Pharmaceutical temptation

We have personally experienced this situation on a few occasions and Edwards presents one in *The M & M Files*.[14] On a follow-up visit from the emergency department, an ophthalmologist discovered that a corneal metallic foreign body was not diagnosed, and that the patient had been self-medicating his eye with a bottle of tetracaine topical anesthetic. After the patient told him that it was prescribed by the ED physician, he decided to call the ED director to file a complaint.

The ED physician stated that he had left the tetracaine next to the patient after the exam but denied giving it to him to use at home. As Edwards points out, leaving a bottle of topical analgesic out is a great temptation for the patient. The patient is in pain, the medicine relieved his pain, the medicine will probably be discarded anyway, and the patient does not have to go to a pharmacy. He also explains the risks with using topical ophthalmic anesthetics at home, which include 'the potential for delayed healing, inadvertent reinjury, and failure to seek appropriate follow-up care.'[15]

Case 7.18 Improper disposal

Another case from Edwards' *The M & M Files* involves a very infrequently used medication.[16] A 29-year-old intoxicated woman came to the ED after a syncopal episode. She was awake on arrival to the ED but became comatose when her mother, her significant other, or the physician entered the room. The nurse handed the physician an ammonium capsule. After he broke the capsule and placed it near her nose, she awoke and tried to attack the doctor and the nurse. During the excitement, the physician did not notice that he had dropped the ammonium capsule.

The physician examined her and ordered routine blood work, which were all unremarkable with the exception of a blood alcohol level of 290 mg/dl. After observing the patient for 3½ hours, the physician decided to honor the patient's request to be discharged. His decision was based on the patient's good social support system, her lack of suicidal thoughts, and her lack of regular alcohol abuse.

Several months later, an attorney for the patient contacted the hospital. He stated that the patient had suffered a physical injury to her thigh resulting from prolonged contact exposure to the ammonium capsule. This injury, he claimed, took over six weeks to heal and required multiple physician visits. The hospital decided to offer a small settlement and an 'adverse outcome' notation was made in the physician's file.

This case is slightly different from the previous case because of two

continued

reasons. The medication used in this case is not a common one. Some physicians may be unaware of the injury that is caused from prolonged contact exposure to it. Secondly, the medication was left in the presence of a patient with a depressed mental status. Besides prolonged contact exposure, the patient could have ingested it, placed it in her eye, or done something else with it.

There are times when textbooks are inaccurate or one reference may not be enough

We have all heard the phrase 'some patients forgot to read the book.' We use this term whenever a patient's symptoms are not classically defined in the textbooks. There are times, however, when patients may have symptoms that are not defined in any textbook or are only found in selective textbooks. We must not forget that clinical symptoms can be very subjective and disease processes can interact with human physiology in various ways.

Case 7.19 The patient 'did not read the book'

Tony Dajer, MD presents his own case, in *Medical Economics*, where a patient's lack of a 'textbook' symptom misguided his physician's treatment decisions.[17] An elderly lady was brought to the ED with the sudden onset of vertigo and vomiting. The physician immediately recalled from his reading the decision pathway for patients with sudden vertigo. He remembered that if a headache is present, there may be a cerebellar hemorrhage and the evaluation will require a head CT. He also read that if there is no headache, the patient just has labyrinthitis.

As he asked the patient this decisive question, he noticed that she was afraid to move her head because any movement would make her vertigo worse. After the patient answered 'no', the physician felt confident with his treatment plan but decided to confirm the patient's response by asking the patient's daughter. After the daughter gave the confirmation, the physician reassured the family. He even felt assured enough to make this a teaching point for his medical student.

The physician was so determined that this patient did not have a serious cause of vertigo that he did not give a second thought to the patient's elevated blood pressure despite no given history of hypertension. He also did not pay too much attention to the fact that his medical student did not examine the patient's cerebellar functioning.

The patient was tried on multiple medications for vertigo without any significant improvement. The physician signed the patient out to another ED physician as 'labyrinthitis' and left for the evening. Upon his return the following morning, he discovered that the patient had stopped breathing a few hours later and could not be resuscitated. He started to wonder whether

continued

the patient died of a heart attack or a cerebellar hemorrhage. Either diagnosis would have represented a missed one because he had not ordered an electrocardiogram or a head CT.

The autopsy report gave the final verdict as a cerebellar hemorrhage. Distraught at missing the diagnosis, the physician went back to review his textbooks. In the one that he had considered as the 'bible' and had read three times, the finding supported his initial belief. It stated that the diagnosis of cerebellar hemorrhages 'should be suspected in any patient with sudden onset of headache, vertigo, vomiting, and ataxia.'[18] Other textbooks that he researched contained similar information. Finally, he was surprised when he stumbled on to an emergency medicine text that stated 'headache, nausea, and vomiting may or may not be present.'[18] So as it stands, this ED physician was in a position that we all probably face at some point in our careers. Despite extensive reading on a subject about which we feel extremely confident, there exists another source somewhere that contains data, in black and white, that suggests that we made an error.

Be careful with patients on Coumadin

Coumadin is a very important drug. It is effective, has many indications, is easy to take, and has prolonged the lives of many patients. Its narrow therapeutic range and the difficulty with maintaining this range, however, have also led to many patient complications on this drug. Consequently, the drug has been a direct or indirect component of numerous medical malpractice lawsuits.

Coumadin is an anticoagulant and is used to thin the blood. It has numerous indications including the prevention of strokes, blood clots, and arterial emboli. Its efficacy can also be affected by many interactions with certain medications and foods. Many patients are not good candidates for the drug (e.g. patients with frequent falls, patients with histories of gastrointestinal bleeding). Lastly, because of the bleeding risk, it can lead to many complications. Whenever you see a patient on Coumadin, always consider whether the complaint is related to the drug and whether the patient is in the therapeutic range of the drug. The following example is one from our clinical practice.

Case 7.20 Add anticoagulant use to the problem list

A 60-year-old man with a history of aortic valve replacement and Coumadin usage presented to our ED after being attacked by a pit bull. He had multiple puncture wounds on his extremities with the most severe one causing a fracture of his right distal ulna. Because he had a significant amount of bleeding from the wounds and his use of Coumadin, we checked his hemoglobin and his prothrombin time. Although we were more concerned about his prothrombin time being prolonged and the difficulty with stopping his bleeding, his prothrombin time returned in the normal range and his bleeding was stopped with pressure.

continued

We called the on-call orthopedist to treat the patient's open fracture. After the orthopedist had treated his wounds, he discharged the patient from the hospital. We were busy tending to other patients in the department and did not see the patient prior to discharge. That night, it struck us that the patient had an artificial heart valve and was not therapeutic on his Coumadin. Although this was an unrelated problem to his ED visit, what if he formed a clot on his valve and had a stroke? This would be bad for him and certainly come back to haunt us because we had ordered his blood work. We drove to the hospital the following day to obtain the patient's demographics. All of his phone numbers were disconnected. We then sent out certified letters to inform him of this problem and called his primary physician to also inform him of this. We hope that the message got to the patient in time but this case certainly demonstrates how a physician must maintain high medical guard and alertness when treating a patient on Coumadin.

Make sure that all of your medical staff introduce themselves to patients

Medical practices may have many different people examining patients. This group includes physician assistants, nurse practitioners, medical students, nurses, etc. The current medical fashions are not as traditional as they have been in the past. We see far fewer physicians with white coats and ties and far fewer nurses with white outfits than in the past. Therefore, it can become confusing to the patient by whom they are being examined.

This type of misunderstanding can be prevented by several techniques. The best and easiest way is to have all personnel introduce themselves when they meet the patient. This ensures that the patient is aware of the capacity that the individual serves. An alternative is to have staff members wear name badges. Badges are not helpful, however, if the patient never reads them. The final method is to have personnel and their positions printed for the patient to read (e.g. letterhead, plaque on wall, etc.). Again, this technique has the same limitations as that of the badges.

In the event of an adverse outcome, a defense is considerably weakened if the patient did not know who treated them.

Case 7.21 Mistaken identity

In Selbst and Korin's *Preventing Malpractice Lawsuits in Pediatric Emergency Medicine*, this confusion contributed to a large settlement.[19] When a five-month-old infant was taken to an urgent care center for a fever she was evaluated by a physician assistant. The child's mother made the assumption that this person was a physician. The child was diagnosed with a viral illness and given no medications.

When the pediatrician evaluated the infant three days later, she found

continued

that the patient had meningitis. This infection left her with moderate mental retardation and cerebral palsy. A lawsuit was filed against the medical center and its physician owner citing failure to properly identify its employees and failure to properly supervise its employees. The plaintiff was awarded $2.5 million.

Chronic problems often require expedient work-ups

Although the above statement may sound counterintuitive, it makes logical sense. Emergency physicians generally regard emergencies as acute problems and chronic problems as ones 'that can wait.' This philosophy has a slight alteration in the office setting. Patients who present with symptoms that have been present for a significant amount of time are likely to have a serious etiology (e.g. cancer). Therefore, although they are not emergencies, they need to be evaluated expediently to minimize morbidity, mortality, and liability.

Case 7.22 How long has this been going on?

Starr presents a case, in *Cortlandt Forum*, where a chronic problem was not worked up expediently. This led to a delay in diagnosis and a large verdict for the plaintiff.[20] A 45-year-old man saw his family practitioner for 15 months of epigastric pain with bloating, belching, and nausea. He had recently developed red blood in his stools on two occasions. His physician attempted to treat him with acidity and indigestion remedies.

After six months, there was no improvement in his symptoms. He was then referred for an upper gastrointestinal series. A radiologist read this report one week later as normal. Months later, the patient was referred to a gastroenterologist. A gastroscopy showed a large fungating mass at the gastroesophageal junction. The patient underwent surgery, chemotherapy, radiation, and died three years later from metastases to the brain. His wife filed a lawsuit against the family practitioner, the radiologist, and the hospital for a delay in diagnosis. The final verdict was for $2.2 million with 62% of the fault attributed to the hospital and the radiologist and 38% of the fault attributed to the family practitioner.

We have participated in numerous physician discussion groups concerning the management of gastroesophageal reflux (GERD) type symptoms through the years. Indeed, many of this patient's symptoms were consistent with GERD. We have learned that this disease is extremely common and that gastric cancers are relatively rare. Therefore, although most physicians would like to see patients with these symptoms get endoscopy early in their treatment regimen, it is not financially feasible. In addition, there are not enough gastroenterologists to accomplish this feat. This patient, however, had the red flags of bleeding and a prolonged course of symptoms. These warning signs warranted a more expedient gastroenterology referral.

References

1 Leinen A and Guldner G (2003) Malpractice or misfortune: we, the jury, find the emergency physician... *EMpulse*. **8**(6): 21–2.
2 Leinen A and Guldner G (2003) Malpractice or misfortune: we, the jury, find the emergency physician... *EMpulse*. **8**(6): 22.
3 Edwards FJ (2002) *The M & M Files: morbidity and mortality rounds in emergency medicine*. Hanley & Belfus Inc., Philadelphia, Pennsylvania, 105–6.
4 Edwards FJ (2002) *The M & M Files: morbidity and mortality rounds in emergency medicine*. Hanley & Belfus Inc., Philadelphia, Pennsylvania, 121–3.
5 Edwards FJ (2002) *The M & M Files: morbidity and mortality rounds in emergency medicine*. Hanley & Belfus Inc., Philadelphia, Pennsylvania, 130–31.
6 Edwards FJ (2002) *The M & M Files: morbidity and mortality rounds in emergency medicine*. Hanley & Belfus Inc., Philadelphia, Pennsylvania, 213–14.
7 Edwards FJ (2002) *The M & M Files: morbidity and mortality rounds in emergency medicine*. Hanley & Belfus Inc., Philadelphia, Pennsylvania, 213.
8 Amsterdam EA, Goldberg RJ, Kelley RE *et al.* (2004) How not to miss commonly overlooked diagnoses. *Patient Care*. **38**(8): 30–37.
9 Rice B (2004) How to neutralize the sympathy factor. *Medical Economics*. **81**(4): 80–82.
10 Rice B (2004) How to neutralize the sympathy factor. *Medical Economics*. **81**(4): 80.
11 Rice B (2004) How to neutralize the sympathy factor. *Medical Economics*. **81**(4): 81.
12 Edwards FJ (2002) *The M & M Files: morbidity and mortality rounds in emergency medicine*. Hanley & Belfus Inc., Philadelphia, Pennsylvania, 158–9.
13 Edwards FJ (2002) *The M & M Files: morbidity and mortality rounds in emergency medicine*. Hanley & Belfus Inc., Philadelphia, Pennsylvania, 159.
14 Edwards FJ (2002) *The M & M Files: morbidity and mortality rounds in emergency medicine*. Hanley & Belfus Inc., Philadelphia, Pennsylvania, 207–8.
15 Edwards FJ (2002) *The M & M Files: morbidity and mortality rounds in emergency medicine*. Hanley & Belfus Inc., Philadelphia, Pennsylvania, 208.
16 Edwards FJ (2002) *The M & M Files: morbidity and mortality rounds in emergency medicine*. Hanley & Belfus Inc., Philadelphia, Pennsylvania, 215–16.
17 Dajer T (2004) Who's to blame? *Medical Economics*. **81**(8): 41–3.
18 Dajer T (2004) Who's to blame? *Medical Economics*. **81**(8): 43.
19 Selbst SM and Korin JB (1999) *Preventing Malpractice Lawsuits in Pediatric Emergency Medicine*. American College of Emergency Physicians, Dallas, Texas, 124.
20 Starr DS (2004) Nonspecific symptoms lead to missed diagnosis. *Cortlandt Forum*. **17**(6): 87–8.

Chapter 8

Things that may go wrong (but are out of your control)

- Equipment failure
- Procedure failures
- Delay in transfers
- Prolonged waiting times
- Consultant is occupied
- Class action medical lawsuits
- New tactics for malpractice lawsuits by attorneys
- Abandonment of insurance companies during lawsuits
- Laboratory error
- Medication error
- Patient non-compliance
- Non-professional expert witnesses and frivolous lawsuits
- Inherent errors of the practice
- The weight factor
- Making judgment decisions that involve risks to the patient
- The lack of equipment and/or facilities
- Problems with housestaff

We felt it would be interesting to include this chapter to remind our readers of the many aspects of medicine of which we have little or no control. It serves as a reminder to us that, regardless of how many years we went to school or spent in clinical training, we are not always the sole determinant of a patient's outcome. Although we cannot give many suggestions on how to control these external factors, we still feel that physicians can practice medicine more defensively if they are aware of these factors.

Equipment failure

Medicine is a highly technological field. We use sophisticated electronic equipment in our daily practices to help us diagnose and treat patients. In fact, some of these electronic equipment have become the 'standard of care' in some areas and are heavily utilized. Examples would be a head CT scan for acute symptoms of stroke to rule out an intracranial bleed, pelvic ultrasound to rule out ectopic pregnancy, and echocardiogram to rule out cardiac tamponade.

This equipment, however, is susceptible to mechanical malfunction in the same manner as any other technological device. Unfortunately, due to their exorbitant costs and their restricted uses, they are much more difficult and timely to replace compared to computers, televisions, etc. Therefore, when a physician needs a vital piece of medical equipment that is not functioning, he arrives at a dilemma with potential legal consequences that may be beyond his control.

Case 8.1 When is it going to be fixed?

Guldner and Leinen describe a case in *EMpulse* of an elderly man who came to the emergency department with left arm and leg weakness.[1] A head CT scan was ordered for the evaluation of possible stroke but was not obtained within the first four hours due to high volume of patients in the emergency department. The emergency physician was then informed that the CT scanner was broken. Two hours later, the repair technicians were unsure of the time needed to complete the repair and the decision was made to transfer the patient to a facility with an operating CT scan. The patient's exam was unchanged at time of transfer but quickly deteriorated in the ambulance en route to the receiving hospital. The CT scan then showed a massive intracranial bleed and the patient endured a complicated course in a nursing care facility and died six months later. The emergency physician and the hospital were found at fault for not obtaining a timely CT scan and a huge monetary settlement was paid on the plaintiff's behalf.

This example is all too common in the emergency department. We formerly worked in an emergency department that had only one CT scanner. Although the scanner was less than one year old, it seemed to be malfunctioning at least once every two weeks. The repair time typically averaged six to eight hours but was occasionally longer. Similar to the mentioned case, the repairman rarely gave us an accurate estimation how long the repair time would be. This uncertainty makes it extremely difficult for the emergency physician to decide whether to hold the patient or transfer him to another facility for a CT scan. To further complicate matters, a transfer to another facility does not guarantee that the patient will receive a CT scan quickly. Other facilities may have their own patients who are waiting for CT scans.

Procedure failures

Procedures, like equipment, are also susceptible to failure. In fact, we like to regard this section as a broader section that encompasses the previous section. This is because the equipments that are used in procedures have their own inherent failure rates, while the physicians who perform these procedures will have their natural complication rates. The natural complication rate is defined as outcomes that are not desirable but consistent and not exceeding the outcomes of other physicians who perform the same procedures. It has no relevance to the clinician's experience or skill.

For example, pneumothorax is a known complication of subclavian vein catheterization. The incidence has been reported to be as high as five incidences in 98 catheterizations.[2] It is an accepted dogma in the medical community that any physician who performs a significant amount of subclavian vein catheterizations will eventually cause a pneumothorax. The occurrence of this complication does not equate with medical malpractice or physician incompetence. We ourselves have also been guilty of this complication. Similarly, tubal ligations also have a known complication of fertility. While some may be attributed to poor physician technique, most occur due to reanastomosis of the tubes, according to our gynecology colleagues. The 'natural' rate of reanastomosis varies with the technique used (from 0–2 pregnancies per 1000 by the Filshie clip method, to six pregnancies per 1000 by the interval laparotomy method).[3] There have been a growing number of lawsuits by women who bear healthy children after having a tubal ligation. A number of these cases have landed settlements against the physician, holding her responsible for the financial expenses of raising the child. Although any particular case may just be the unfortunate and unpreventable outcome of the procedure, to the jury and to the woman involved it is that woman's devastating emotional and financial loss. Plaintiff attorneys are aware of the emotions involved and will dramatize them to the best of their ability.

Case 8.2 Road left unexplored

We found a story printed in the *Physicians Financial News* especially interesting.[4] This event occurred in Australia and involved a surgeon who was found guilty of medical negligence for a failed sterilization procedure. The physician involved performed a left tubal ligation on a patient for sterilization after she had informed him that she had her right fallopian tube removed years earlier during an appendectomy. Five years later, the patient had a healthy son and it was discovered that her right fallopian tube was never removed. Although the case was not specific as to how the lady became fertile, it is assumed that it was due to the remaining right fallopian tube. She successfully sued the physician and was awarded more than $133 000. She also received $70 000 as financial compensation to raise her son.

This case illustrates two interesting legal issues. The patient informed her physician that her right fallopian tube had already been removed. In the same manner that the public expects their physicians to be honest to them, should physicians not expect the same from their patients? If the surgeon had explored the patient's right abdomen to see if the tube had actually been removed, would this have been regarded as battery for violating a part of the body that the patient did not feel needed to be explored (or given consent for)? If the physician had made an attempt at obtaining records to confirm the previous surgery, he would have helped his legal defense. Alternatively, it might have been beneficial to state on the consent form that the patient was only consenting to removal of the left fallopian tube. Regardless of whether these things were done, the patient's history makes the verdict of this case difficult to understand in the medical community.

The second issue is when and how we decide to hold physicians responsible for complications that could be natural consequences of a procedure. If the trend is to hold physicians at fault the majority of the time, there will certainly be a decrease in the number of physicians performing the procedure. Patients will suffer due to longer waits and narrower selection of physicians, while physicians will suffer due to loss of income. Failures are inherent in every contraceptive method. Failure rates of birth control pills and condoms are well published.

Delay in transfers

Transfers are extremely time-consuming because they require numerous inter-active phone calls between the facilities involved. There must be direct contact by physician to physician and an accepting physician must be obtained. Once there is an accepting physician, the transfer must be approved by the nursing supervisor concerning bed availability. Then, a conversation between the involved parties regarding the mode of transportation must be made. We have had the most difficulty with transferring patients to specialty centers that are more than fifty miles away. Turf battles often ensue between cities concerning who should send the helicopter or ambulance. Furthermore, distant transportation is often delayed or declined in inclement weather. Even transfers within the same city often take hours while awaiting the arrival of the local ambulance. After these details are finalized, all paperwork must be copied, transferred forms filled out completely, X-rays copied, and the sending physician must perform her final exam. Finally, a direct transfer report must be made from nurse to nurse. As anyone can probably conjecture, in the time it takes to perform all of these duties, most defects in the CT scanner could probably be fixed. Hence, the decision for the emergency physician to transfer or keep is not always as clear as plaintiff attorneys claim it to be in court.

Prolonged waiting times

Waiting times are becoming an increasing problem in the primary care office but have always been a major dilemma for emergency departments. In an article from *American Medical News* it is reported that 'more than 107 million people sought care in the nation's 4045 hospital emergency departments in 2001.'[5] This is an average of over three patients per hour seen in each emergency depart-ment. This number, however, exceeds the American College of Emergency Physicians recommendations of less than two and a half patients seen per hour per physician for best quality of care. Hence, for the majority of emergency departments that have single physician coverage, waiting times will be longer than expected. Given these statistics, it is not hard to see that some of us are inherently practicing medicine with increased liability.

It is every emergency physician's nightmare to have three or four ambulances containing patients with chest pain arrive simultaneously. Who do you decide to see first? What about the multiple trauma scenarios? How about the critical care patient that requires more than thirty minutes of one-to-one care? These are all situations where even the greatest and fastest doctors in the world may be faulted for delayed care resulting in adverse outcomes.

Although these situations are largely not under our control, they are high liability situations, not immune from legal action, and just as difficult to defend in court. You are not likely to draw any sympathy from the judge or jurors about how busy you were that day or how many simultaneous emergencies you had at the moment in question. This is because of several reasons. First, it is difficult to show documentation years later of how hectic that day was for you or whose life you were saving when the patient in question was not getting treated. Second, judges and jurors have not likely spent a day in a busy emergency department and will have difficulty relating to your plea. Finally, it is irrelevant that you were saving someone's life; the courtroom's concern is with the damage to the patient in question. Our profession is unlike law, teaching, etc. where you can make people wait and cause them no physical harm.

Case 8.3 I am tired of waiting

Albert writes about a physician who was sued by his patient for the patient's prolonged wait time.[6] The physician received a phone call from one of his patients who requested an add-on appointment for a pain medication injection. Although the physician's schedule was full that day, he agreed to see the patient since the patient was leaving for a vacation the following day. The physician's day was busier than he had anticipated and the patient ended up waiting in his office for three hours before deciding to leave without seeing the physician. The patient, subsequently, filed a lawsuit for $5000 as compensation for his lost time. The courts awarded the patient $250.

We felt that the court's handling of the above case was inappropriate for several reasons. It may set a precedent for future medical cases of prolonged wait times. As we discussed earlier in this section, prolonged wait times are often not a fault of the physician and are largely a problem of the American (and probably universal) medical system. How many patients can answer that they have never had to wait to see a doctor? A better question is how many people can testify to having never had to wait at any particular business? We have had to wait for over 24 hours over the anticipated completion time to have our automobiles serviced and hours over our appointment time to renew our driver's licenses. However, because the mechanic and the clerk at the driver's license office are not considered 'deep pockets', they are rarely included in lawsuits.

Case 8.4 Racing against the clock

In an excellent example of delayed care in the emergency department from *The M & M Files*, Edwards writes about a 47-year-old female who presented after suddenly developing chest pressure and shortness of breath while watching television.[7] She had no prior medical history and had her ankle in a cast from a fracture that she suffered two weeks ago. On presentation

continued

to the ED, she was cyanotic, diaphoretic, tachycardic, hypotensive, and gasping for air. Her arterial blood gas revealed that she was hypoxic and hyperventilating.

As the emergency physician was waiting for the chest X-ray, he was also evaluating a patient with suspected intra-abdominal injuries from a motor vehicle accident and another patient with an active myocardial infarction. He returned to the shortness of breath patient 10 minutes later to find that she had become unconscious with unpalpable pulses. She was immediately intubated and cardiopulmonary resuscitation was attempted for 45 minutes to no avail. The etiology of her death at autopsy was a massive pulmonary embolism. Her 'husband contacted the state health department and an attorney, concerned over why the patient had not been given a "clot buster" when she first arrived' (9, 41). Although the ED physician probably had little doubt as to the cause of this unfortunate lady's shortness of breath, he was, nevertheless, faulted for not immediately intubating this patient and for not considering the use of fibrinolytic agents. This case highlights the difficulty of not making perfect decisions when a physician is presented with multiple critical patients simultaneously. The physician's goal is to make decisions that will obtain the best outcome for all of her patients at that moment. The court's concern, however, is only with the patient that suffered the adverse outcome and does not consider the outcomes of the other patients that were treated at the same time.

As a final note, there are plaintiff attorneys who will try to exploit this problem to boost their business. One attorney in a large Florida city advertises on a large billboard that you should call him if your wait time in the emergency department is long. Our view is that prolonged waiting times in the emergency department are the norm (look at the numbers above) due to ED overcrowding rather than the exception. It is not a problem of the physician, the hospital, the city, or the state. It is a national problem and is tied to our healthcare system. There are no easy solutions and the physicians and hospitals should not, in general, be held responsible.

Consultant is occupied

There are two hospitals in the town where we practice. Within a radius of 50 miles of our town are much smaller communities with a relative dearth of medical specialists. Therefore, our specialty consultants are frequently not only on call for both hospitals on the same night but are also asked to accept care from outlying physicians in the smaller communities. Hence, it is inevitable that they will be asked to see multiple emergency patients simultaneously. In the event that the consultant is in the middle of a procedure (e.g. heart surgery), the wait for another patient could become extensive. Similar to the previous discussions, it becomes the emergency physician's responsibility to keep the waiting patient stable or seek alternative specialist evaluation (e.g. transfer to another facility, or asking a specialist who is not on call). Although the scope of the ED physician's control of the situation is limited, she will likely be attached to any lawsuit should the patient's condition deteriorate while she is waiting for the consultant's arrival.

An alternative approach for managing the emergency patient when the consultant is occupied is to seek the assistance of a consultant from another medical specialty. For example, if a patient with chest pain requires admission but the cardiologist is tied up in the catheterization laboratory, the medical internist on call could be asked to see and admit the patient. The specialists occasionally make this request to the ED physicians. This approach, however, can be a double-edged sword in terms of medical liability. If the emergency physician is occupied in the department with several critical patients at the same time, having the internist assume care of an unstable angina patient versus sharing your attention to this patient's needs with other critical patients in the department may lead to the patient's best outcome. From the other perspective, however, if the patient suffers a massive myocardial infarction while under the care of the internist, the plaintiff attorneys will not hesitate to fault the emergency physician for placing the patient under substandard medical care.

Class action medical lawsuits

Physicians are increasingly being named in class action lawsuits against drug companies. We were at a malpractice lecture at the 2003 American Academy of Family Physicians Annual Assembly and this was a surprisingly common problem among our colleagues. In many cases, the physician's patients were unaware that their physician was named in their suits. This omission of information made for an awkward situation when the physician had to address the problem with his or her patient. The physician is uneasy because most of us cannot continue to care for patients who are suing us, because any conversation that we continue to have with them may be used against us in court. The patients also feel uneasy because many are surprised and have had congenial relationships with their physicians for many years. Many patients will even state that they would have never signed their name to the lawsuit had they known that their physician was part of the defense. Attorneys will strategically omit physician names in order to get more patients to sign on to the lawsuit.

In an article concerning class action lawsuits in *Medical Economics*, Pennachio states that 'law firms troll for plaintiffs for these suits. If you go to www.plaintiffdirectmail.com, you'll get an inkling of how easy it is for attorneys to build a class.'[8] The website also contains data of over 60 drugs and a database of over 30 000 000 people who it claims have been harmed by these drugs.[8] The company reveals that it obtains its information from consumer surveys.[8] Once the attorneys attract their plaintiffs to a class action lawsuit, they impose a time limit in which the plaintiff can withdraw their participation. This technique is used by the attorneys with the hope that any patient who does not wish to sue his or her private physician will discover their private physician's involvement at a point that is beyond the limit for participation withdrawal.

Case 8.5 Products we hate to see go

Elizabeth Connell, MD, in *Family Practice News*, talks about how frivolous lawsuits have devastated the field of reproductive medical technology.[9] These frivolous lawsuits are similar to class action lawsuits in the sense that they involve one particular product but not true class action lawsuits because they are filed independently for each product. Bendectin, the only drug that was ever developed for nausea and vomiting specifically related to pregnancy, was pulled from the market in 1983. The withdrawal was due to a high number of claims that the drug was responsible for birth defects. These claims, however, were not verified by convincing scientific data.

A similar fate resulted for two good intrauterine devices in the 1980s, the Copper-7 and the Tatum-T. Lawsuits for these products were based on the occurrence of pelvic infections in their users. Again, there was no convincing data and the manufacturers were winning most of the lawsuits. They still decided to pull the products from the market, however, because of increasing legal defense costs. Now, in 2004, we still have to warn patients with intrauterine devices of the increased risk of pelvic infections. Have these lawsuits resulted in better and safer products?

Other examples that Dr Connell mentions include the six-rod Norplant contraceptive and gel-filled silicone implants. Both of these products contain silicone, a product that has long been the subject of a legal claim that it causes autoimmune disease. Again, Dr Connell states that there has been no legal proof of this cause-and-effect phenomenon. She also points out that the products mentioned in the preceding paragraphs along with the six-rod Norplant contraceptive were all pulled from the market without ever losing their FDA approval status.

New tactics for malpractice lawsuits by attorneys

Attorneys are finding new ways to increase physician responsibility and liability in order for them to file more lawsuits.

Case 8.6 Get rich schemes

Tanya Albert, in *American Medical News*, writes an excellent article highlighting some of these new tactics.[10] She notes that the family of a man in Ohio was awarded $3.5 million after he had died of a heart attack. The award was not for the conventional reasons of missed diagnosis, delayed treatment, or incorrect treatment. Rather, the award was because the treating physician did not 'do enough to help the man lose weight and stop smoking.'[10] Although the case is being appealed, the verdict is frightening for physicians because we know that some patients will not give up smoking or lose weight if their life depends on it (as it did in this case). The argument is that there are now medical advances for smoking cessation

continued

and weight loss. However, most physicians, and the public for that matter, will probably agree that they are also social problems in addition to medical problems. Physicians can only help so much and patients need to assume some responsibility for their own health.

Case 8.7 Right of free enterprise

The article also discusses the interesting case of a Florida resident who filed a lawsuit against a hospital and some of its physicians for not referring her to another local hospital to have a tumor removed.[10] She claimed that the other hospital performed more of these procedures than the hospital where she was treated and, therefore, it was the treating hospital's obligation to refer her. We do not agree with this reasoning for a couple of reasons. The first is that it was never a question of whether the treating hospital had physicians certified to perform the given procedure. In the medical field, there is not a clear distinction between two physicians who are equally certified, and performing more procedures does not necessarily equate to being more skilled. The former statement is supported by EMTALA (Emergency Medical Treatment and Active Labor Act) guidelines, which require a hospital to perform a certain procedure if it has a certified physician on staff capable of performing that procedure. The guidelines also prevent a hospital from dumping the procedure onto another hospital because the other hospital has more trained physicians. Second, medicine is also a business that seeks to keep its own customers. Does a mechanic tell you that he can do the repair but he is going to refer you to the automobile shop down the street because they have repaired more cars? Maybe we should ask the plaintiff attorney who instigated this lawsuit if he has ever referred a lawsuit to a more experienced attorney at another firm. It is partly the responsibility of the patient to ask about the physician's experience and whether there are more experienced physicians in the area. We strongly believe that most physicians would give their patient an honest answer and would be happy to refer the patient at her request. In any event, the above patient had a complicated course since her surgery and has required numerous follow-up surgeries. The case is scheduled to go to trial soon.

Case 8.8 Burden of responsibility

Starr presents a case in *Cortlandt Forum* where plaintiff attorneys are now finding ways to hold physicians liable for patient non-compliance.[11] The case involves a family practitioner and his treatment of a teenager for depression. The young man was diagnosed with depression and attention deficit disorder when he was a high school senior. He was started on medications for both at this time and referred to a counselor. Despite the physician's encouragement (although documentation of this was not in the

continued

chart), the patient abandoned his therapist over the next year. He had agreed to go to another therapist but never did so. Instead, he continued to take the medications and told his doctor that his depression was getting worse and that he had developed some suicidal ideations.

The family practitioner then moved his practice thousands of miles away. When the patient tried to contact his old office to talk to him, he was told that 'he no longer works here.' The patient ceased his efforts at contacting his physician after several days. During the next month, he repeatedly rehearsed his suicide plan and finally shot himself in the face. The suicide attempt was unsuccessful but left him with blindness and permanent disfigurement.

The patient and his family filed a lawsuit against the family physician. They contend that the patient should have been referred to a psychiatrist when his depression was worsening. They also claim that the physician did not alter his therapy when it was needed and did not take the patient's suicidal ideations seriously. The physician, in contrast, said that he had recommended psychiatric counseling on multiple occasions and felt that the suicide was largely the patient's fault for not finding help after he had moved away.

During trial, the defense was largely based on the patient's non-compliance in counseling therapy whereas the plaintiff attorney faulted the physician for not being aggressive enough with getting the patient help. Although the plaintiff was seeking $10 million in damages, the verdict was for $5.5 million, with 45% of the liability to the patient and 55% of the liability to the physician. Therefore, the final verdict was for over $3 million against the physician.

In the past, physicians have generally been immune to medical malpractice when patient compliance is an issue. As Starr points out, plaintiff attorneys have now become skilled at convincing jurors that the lack of patient compliance is a result of physician negligence.[12] Please see the further discussion in the section on 'Patient non-compliance' below. The other interesting legal issue about this case is that of the comparative fault statutes that many states have now adopted.[12] Court rulings are no longer all-or-nothing as they were in the past. Rather, fault is given as a percentage and the physician has to be deemed liable for greater than 50% fault for damages to be awarded based on the percentages.

The last new strategy among attorneys has to do with tort reform. Due to the new laws in many states placing a cap on non-economic damages, plaintiff attorneys are looking for other avenues to draw large gains. This has led to an increased frequency of hospitals and surgical/medical centers being named in lawsuits along with physicians. Although this may appear to benefit physicians because they are named in lawsuits less often it also makes it more difficult for physicians to get on hospital staff. Plaintiff attorneys have frequently charged hospitals with inadequate credentialing in order to name hospitals in lawsuits. Even for physicians who have a 'clean' record, it may take months to get hospital privileges.

Abandonment of insurance companies during lawsuits

Insurance companies are first and foremost businesses. They exist to make money just like any other business. When a lawsuit takes place, the insurance company is responsible for financing the physician's defense as well as any settlement or award from the suit. Therefore, the extent of the suit that the insurance company wishes to undertake is sometimes influenced by the potential of winning the case and the estimated cost of defending the case. For example, a case that has obvious or likely medical malpractice involved will probably cause the insurance company to settle before going to court in order to minimize the estimated payout. They are aware that the longer a suit continues, the more the amount of money invested by both parties will increase. Consequently, the plaintiff attorney will request a larger award. It has also been published that judges will take the plaintiff attorney's expenses into consideration when determining the size of the award. By settling the case early, the company also avoids a large defense team bill. Even if a case is deemed worthy of trial, it may be settled if the insurance company determines that it may persist for a lengthy duration with an accompanying astronomical cost for the defense attorney. Hence, the insurance company's objectives are not always consistent with that of the physician that it insures. The defense attorney, who is usually hired by the insurance company, may also not have consistent objectives with that of the physician that he represents. Some insurance companies and defense attorneys, however, will have a clause stating that no decision during the suit will be made without the physician's approval.

Case 8.9 Never had a chance

Starr presents another case in *Cortlandt Forum*, which we strongly believe was trial-worthy but was, nevertheless, settled against the physician.[13] A 26-year-old man went to see his family physician for an injury to his leg. The injury occurred after he had jumped onto a boat deck and landed on a wineglass. The glass had shattered and one of the pieces cut his leg just behind the lateral malleolus. The physician examined the patient's ankle and wound and did not find any significant injuries. He therefore cleaned the wound, sutured it, and referred the patient to an orthopedist.

The patient followed up with the orthopedist two weeks later. The wound was healing well and the musculoskeletal examination of the ankle was normal. The orthopedist released the patient and instructed him to return as needed. The man returned to work and participation in lacrosse. Shortly later, he felt weakness in his right calf during a game. This led him to see a sports medicine doctor. This physician made the diagnosis of a complete tear of the posterior tibial tendon, which he felt would need a graft repair.

The patient obtained an attorney who filed a lawsuit against the family physician for missing the tendon tear. During the almost two years of pretrial discovery, the defense claimed that the patient could not have anything more than a partial tear because there was no functional deficit during the initial exam. This claim was well supported by the orthopedist's exam two

continued

weeks later. We believe that the plaintiff attorney knew that he could not provide any objective data to support his claim. Furthermore, the patient returned to active sport activities and could have had a second injury that was completely unrelated to the first. The plaintiff attorney wisely made an offer to settle. Although the defense team had an excellent chance of winning this case, several factors led them to settle for $31 000. This amount probably did little more for the patient than offset two years of legal bills. For the physician, however, this settlement meant a report of malpractice to the National Practitioner's Data Bank and a black mark on his career.

Starr points out several factors why the insurance company decided to settle in this case. 'The company representative at trial felt that the patient's loss of athletic activity made him a sympathetic witness. Furthermore, the trial was held in an area known for its plaintiff sympathies. Finally, the plaintiff lawyer was willing to accept a settlement amount that essentially represented his cost of doing business.'[14] Remember that the insurance company will not lose any sleep over the fact that their physician has received a black mark. Instead, they will be relieved over the money they saved from not paying out a huge award (or defense cost). They can also raise the physician's insurance premiums because of the claim that is made. Does all of this sometimes make physicians wonder just who exactly is on their side? As we can see, all of these factors are, for the most part, out of our control. The only recommendation in this case that we can give is to try to buy malpractice insurance from a company that has a good track record at fighting claims and allows the physician to play an active role in the claim.

Case 8.10 Who do you work for?

In the book *Law For Physicians: an overview of medical legal issues*, published by the American Medical Association, it is discussed that it is also import-ant to find out who is the employer of your defense attorney.[15] The authors note that defense attorneys who are employed by the insurance company may not be able to be impartial to the policyholder. This occurs when the attorney discovers confidential information in his representation of the physician that may be used by the insurance company to deny the physician coverage. This conflict of interest would not be present if an independent attorney represents the physician. The authors report a recent case in Maryland where this exact situation occurred (*Medical Mut Liab Ins Soc of Maryland v Miller*, 451 A2d 930 (1982)).[15] After the physician spent a significant amount of money and time (months away from work) to file a lawsuit against his insurance company, he finally succeeded in obtaining coverage.

Laboratory error

Laboratory machines are operated by technicians and are susceptible to human error. In addition, laboratory machines are not always infallible and specimens are sometimes mislabeled. We previously discussed the patient with chest pain who had elevated cardiac enzymes (i.e. CPK, Troponin I) and was treated for acute myocardial infarction with anticoagulants only to find the next day that the enzymes were from another patient's blood specimen. This was discovered when his cardiac enzymes the following day returned to normal. Errors such as these can be minimized by quality and assurance reviews and by implementing check measures throughout the data analysis. However, they will never be totally eliminated due to the natural acceptable element of human and machine error.

Case 8.11 Confused with someone else

The following case by Wear-Finkle in *Medicolegal Issues in Clinical Practice* illustrates the extensive damage that laboratory errors can create.[16] After an internist had informed a lady that she had syphilis (from the results of a lab), he encouraged her to inform her husband so that they could both be treated. The couple each believed that the other was unfaithful and subsequently got a divorce. The laboratory informed the internist that the result was an error two years later. The patient was outraged at hearing this from her physician. The patient's ex-husband then filed a lawsuit against the doctor and the lab company.

Physicians can do their part in reducing laboratory errors by reviewing every lab personally and signing off on it. It also helps to discuss with the laboratory technician before ordering particular labs to ensure the proper collection and order of the lab (e.g. which tubes to place joint aspirated fluid into). Inform the laboratory technician if you notice any unusual trends in your labs over a particular period (e.g. all potassium levels seem to be high for a particular day).

Medication error

We have discussed in other sections of this book where physicians can make medication errors. Physicians, however, only represent one subset of healthcare professionals who may make medication errors. The pharmacist may incorrectly fill a prescription or order. The pharmacy clerk or technician may dispense or deliver the incorrect medication. Furthermore, medicine may be stocked in the wrong space of the pyxis (medicine cart). Finally, the nurse that administers the medicine may make a mistake.

Case 8.12 More is not better

Edwards presents a case, in *The M & M Files*, where a nurse mistakenly administered an excessive dose of a dangerous medication.[17] A physician had ordered a 5000 unit bolus of heparin for a patient with thrombophlebitis of the leg. The nurse used the more concentrated heparin that is used for flushes and consequently gave the patient 40 000 units of heparin. Fortunately, she discovered and informed the physician immediately and protamine sulfate was given to the patient. With the exception of transient gross hematuria, the patient suffered no long-term complications.

Case 8.13 Putting things in the correct place

Merry and Smith discuss a case in *Errors, Medicine, and the Law* where a drug error led to a patient's death.[18] This case involves an anesthesiologist from New Zealand. At the completion of an operation, the patient was awakening from her general anesthesia when she began biting down on her endotracheal tube. The biting prevented the patient from receiving any oxygen and she quickly developed cyanosis. The surgeon and scrub nurse had already left the operating suite and the anesthesiologist was left with an inexperienced nurse.

The physician requested the analeptic drug, Dopram, and was given a medicine from the drawer labeled as Dopram. Tragically, someone had made the error of placing the drug dopamine into this drawer. After administering this incorrect medicine to the patient, she went into cardiac arrest. The resuscitation was successful but there was irreversible brain damage and the patient died shortly afterwards. The physician reported this incident immediately and this acknowledgement prevented him from receiving a conviction for manslaughter. He was, however, found guilty of medical negligence as the plaintiff attorney argued that the physician should have never given the medicine without checking it. Although this argument is correct and not debatable, it is sometimes difficult to implement this practice when a patient is quickly decompensating in front of you.

Some medications are prone to administration errors and often require an experienced supervisor. One example would be the rapid push of adenosine for supraventricular tachycardia. Another would be the administration of epinephrine. Epinephrine has the diverse ability to be administered intramuscularly, subcutaneously, intravenously, and by nebulizer. It also has a broad range of indications including: arrhythmias, bronchospasms, anaphylaxis, cardiac arrest, and preterm labor. Unfortunately, the different concentrations and different routes of epinephrine administration can sometimes cause confusion and lead to medication errors.

Case 8.14 Watch over carefully

A 34-year-old woman came to the ED after eating a seafood salad. She had a shrimp allergy and did not know that it was present in the salad. She had no past medical history and did not smoke cigarettes. On presentation, her lungs were extremely tight with wheezing and an oxygen saturation of 90% on room air.

The patient's electrocardiogram showed normal sinus rhythm and no acute changes. The emergency physician ordered a subcutaneous injection of epinephrine, intravenous SoluMedrol, intravenous diphenhydramine, and an albuterol nebulizer treatment. He proceeded to evaluate another patient. The patient's nurse drew up the ordered medications from the pyxis. Although she had been a nurse for a few years, she had never administered epinephrine by a route other than intravenously. Her experience with epinephrine use was limited to treating patients with cardiac arrest.

As she went into the patient's room to administer the medications, she had the presumption that all of the medications were going to be given intravenously. Shortly after she gave the epinephrine to the patient intravenously, the patient complained of worsening chest pain. A repeat electrocardiogram showed t wave inversions consistent with ischemia. Her cardiac enzymes also showed subsequent damage to the heart. The dosage of epinephrine given was too much intravenously for the patient's heart to tolerate. A settlement was made to the patient by the hospital.

Unfortunately, mistakes like this one are not as rare as one might believe. We have seen three instances in our career of epinephrine given mistakenly by the intravenous route. Most of these mistakes are not noticed because they do not cause any permanent morbidity or mortality. In fact, many do not cause any symptoms at all. However, recognizing that medication errors like these can cause severe injuries gives us the opportunity to supervise the medications' administration.

Patient non-compliance

Although we must sometimes blame ourselves for patient non-compliance because of inadequate or incomplete instructions, there remains a significant percentage of patients who will simply disregard your instructions. Numerous factors may play a role in this non-compliance. Patients may not be able to afford to see the follow-up physician or buy the necessary medicines. They may be turned away due to their insurance or due to a lack of an opening in the physician's schedule. Some patients do not have the transportation while others lack the education to comprehend their discharge instructions.

In the primary care setting, patients often stop taking their chronic medications once they are feeling better. Getting patients to stay up to date with their health maintenance and cancer screening has always been a challenge for the primary care provider. Finally, primary care patients frequently have multiple medical problems and multiple medications, both of which may contribute to suboptimal compliance.

It is obvious that patient non-compliance, regardless of the cause, can lead to adverse outcomes. Although physicians have little control of their patient's compliance and will not be faulted the majority of the time, physicians should still be careful with their documentation because of expectations of physicians to supervise their patients' actions in some instances. This particularly applies to elderly patients who live alone, developmentally delayed patients, homeless patients, and intoxicated patients. Admitting physicians sometimes get frustrated with emergency physicians for admissions that are made largely for social purposes. However, from a medical-legal standpoint, if a patient or his or her family requests admission and is refused because the patient does not need it medically, the emergency physician may still be found at fault if the patient's condition worsens whether they follow their instructions or not.

Case 8.15 If he would have followed instructions

We were named in a suit a few years ago by a very non-compliant patient. The patient was a heavy smoker and saw us after he hit his toe on a coffee table. X-rays were negative and he was treated for a contusion. He did not take the medicines prescribed for him. He returned to the clinic twice in the next two weeks as the skin started to break down on his toe. He was prescribed antibiotics and referred to podiatry three times and told to stop smoking. He did not comply with any of these recommendations. Two months later, he chose his own podiatrist and presented with an open wound with bone exposed. His podiatrist did not recognize this as clinical osteomyelitis and did not offer him intravenous antibiotics. Instead, he performed surgical debridement of the wound and placed him on oral antibiotics and did not tell him to stop smoking.

Not surprisingly, the podiatrist's malpractice led the wound's infection to become progressively worse. As the patient continued to smoke heavily, he was discovered to have vascular disease and underwent a bypass graft on the involved leg. The vascular surgeon was optimistic about saving the patient's toe with the surgery but the podiatrist involved did not adhere to this advice and amputated the patient's toe two months later against the vascular surgeon's wishes. The patient then decided to file suit and the podiatrist convinced him to name all of the prior physicians. The podiatrist offered to become the patient's expert witness in order to cover up his own malpractice.

The case dragged on for over two years and depositions were made on both sides. We testified at deposition that the patient was non-compliant in not taking his prescribed medications, not following through with specialist appointments as scheduled (he missed over 10 scheduled appointments with podiatry and vascular surgery), and for continuing to smoke despite admonitions from over five different physicians (his own podiatrist excluded). We also pointed out the podiatrist's malpractice in not recognizing clinical osteomyelitis, his failure to treat it aggressively, and his engagement in ill-advised surgery. The case was finally dropped after the review of all the depositions.

As we discussed above, patient non-compliance is no longer the saving grace for physicians it once was. As Starr points out, we have developed and incorporated computer technology into our patient record keeping and are now able to track the patient's medical treatment with extreme precision. Remember the old saying, however, that 'with power comes responsibility.' Here, the responsibility is to ensure patient compliance because the patient may be making an impaired judgment. Ensuring compliance also becomes especially important when fatality may be an end result. Finally, jurors and courts do not look favorably on physicians who do not make a legitimate effort at transferring patient care after closing their practice. This may be regarded in some courts as patient abandonment.

Non-professional expert witnesses and frivolous lawsuits

We have all read about the type of physician that plaintiff attorneys use as expert witnesses. Some are considered 'hired hands' and do not practice clinical medicine. Instead they advertise their services over the internet and travel around the country testifying for plaintiffs only. These individuals, by their nature, do not represent good physicians or good witnesses. We do not see how a physician can be a good clinician if he does not practice clinical medicine. Second, if you do not practice clinical medicine, how can you testify as to the standard of care when you are not actively practicing it? Lastly, standards of care can vary in different areas; therefore, how can one person travel outside of their practice area and give statements as to how medicine should be practiced in another area?

Case 8.16 Will say anything for money

Some expert witnesses will agree to testify even before reviewing the charts of the case. We were once surprised to look in our mailbox and find an intent for initiating lawsuit concerning a case that occurred in a hospital 50 miles from where we lived (and in which we had never practiced). The letter had a written affidavit from a female emergency physician in Miami stating that our emergency care of a pediatric patient (who was admitted and later died in the intensive care unit) was inadequate. This physician swore on oath that she had thoroughly reviewed the charts and that she clearly found fault in our actions. We were perplexed with this letter because we did not have any recollection of a pediatric patient dying at our facility (we did not admit pediatric patients at our facility). Furthermore, we did not work at this outlying hospital.

After we obtained the records ourselves, we discovered that we had seen this patient four months prior to the patient's visit to the outlying hospital. We had treated the patient for upper respiratory complaints that had no relevance to the child's fatal illness at the outlying hospital four months later. The expert witness did not bother to note the signature from the emergency hospital from the visit in question but had read our signature from the emergency visit at our hospital. When we informed the plaintiff

---

continued

attorneys of this *faux pas*, they were quick to apologize by phone and in writing. They stated, however, that we should treasure the letter of apology because it was the first one that they have sent in 15 years. It has been almost three years, however, and we have still not received an apology from the emergency physician who served as the expert witness. After receiving support and assistance from leaders in the Florida College of Emergency Physicians, we wrote letters to our state health agency to try to ban this physician from further testifying but our letters were unanswered.

Our example above of the podiatrist who served as an expert witness against us also raised some other questions regarding the qualifications of an expert witness. Our defense lawyer questioned whether a podiatrist could testify against a medical problem in our state but the case was dropped before we ever obtained a definitive answer. In addition, it was later discovered that this podiatrist had a felony criminal record that was ignored by the plaintiff attorney. Finally, his relationship with the patient should have prevented him from making an impartial expert opinion.

Some physicians have taken similar actions from plaintiff attorneys more seriously than we have.

Case 8.17 Fighting back

Robert Lowes presents a case in *Medical Economics* where two physicians fought back against a prominent attorney for filing a frivolous lawsuit.[19] The case involved a 58-year-old man who presented to the ED and was admitted for symptoms that were later diagnosed as an ischemic stroke. The man died a few days later after being transferred to another facility.

The plaintiff attorney obtained the patient's chart and found that Propulsid was listed as one of his current medications. The lawyer's adrenaline started to flow because he knew that there were a number of lawsuits against the company that produced Propulsid due to its association in studies with arrhythmias and deaths. In fact, the company had pulled the medication off the market approximately one year after the patient had died and also had to deal with a $100 million verdict in Mississippi a year after the drug was pulled. Despite the lack of documentation in the patient's chart of any physician prescribing Propulsid during his stay and comments in the chart that the patient had been off the drug two weeks before coming to the hospital, the attorney filed a shotgun lawsuit on behalf of the patient's widow just a few days prior to the statute of limitations.

The suit named the drug company, the hospital, a nurse practitioner, and eight physicians. The ED physician and the admitting internist were two of the physicians. The main basis of the suit was the accusation that the hospital and the physicians prescribed a dangerous drug, Propulsid, to the patient. Although there were no specifics as to who prescribed the drug, and the connection of this drug to the patient's death, the attorney was just

continued

hoping to get the legal action instigated before the deadline and then sort things out later.

The ED physician and the admitting internist requested separate court motions to investigate the attorney's frivolous claim. In response, the attorney immediately asked that the suit be dropped. He claimed that his action was in response to the wish of the patient's widow. Two other local doctors confirmed that the same attorney had also hit them with frivolous suits. A judge subsequently fined the attorney $50 000 to deter him from further similar activities.

Case 8.18 Turning the tables

We read about another physician in *American Medical News* who had taken matters into her own hands.[20] Julie McCammon, MD, was suing the West Virginia Trial Lawyers Association for engaging in frivolous lawsuits against physicians in West Virginia. She herself had a frivolous lawsuit against her dropped in 1999. She claimed, however, that the majority of frivolous law-suits demand defense expenditure by the insurance company before they are dropped. This, in turn, has been a major factor in increasing insurance premiums in West Virginia. 'Her list of grievances includes: economic loss, professional limitations, emotional distress, mental anguish, and other economic damages.'[21] The judge, who was married to a trial lawyer, dismissed the case but Dr McCammon was appealing the decision. Dr McCammon pointed out that 29% of the lawsuits filed in West Virginia during the past decade were eventually dropped but still required defense spending from the insurance companies.

Tanya Albert, in *American Medical News*, reports a story concerning the impact of frivolous lawsuits on the healthcare system.[22] The article stated that frivolous lawsuits that are eventually dismissed cost 'insurance companies thousands of dollars to defend.'[23] This in turn, increased the cost of medical liability insurance and has forced some physicians to retire, move to another area, or go without insurance. The article also points out that Ohio physicians have become enraged at the 'shotgun' approach by plaintiff attorneys of naming every physician on the chart. In some instances, physicians were named even though their names were not on the chart (similar to our case above). Ohio State Medical Association has responded by forming the Frivolous Lawsuit Committee to whom physicians can report frivolous lawsuits.

Case 8.19 Frivolous but damaging

An example of the impact that a frivolous lawsuit can have on a physician's career is given in the same article. An Ohio intensivist was named in a lawsuit after she had seen a patient for the first time as the patient was

continued

coding. A patient with a history of diabetes and coronary artery disease was transferred by helicopter to the physician's facility for vascular insufficiency. The physician was called to see the patient in the intensive care unit after the patient had gone into cardiac arrest. She was involved with the patient for 15 minutes before the patient died. Nevertheless, she was one of 23 physicians that were later named in a lawsuit on the patient's behalf.

After 17 months, six motions, and a deposition, the case against her was finally dropped. The damage of the lawsuit to her career, however, was irrevocable. She was named in another lawsuit and was eventually dropped from that one also. Her insurer refused to renew her contract when her liability insurance came up for renewal. She and her partners had to switch to a new company with a much more expensive premium and the requirement that she pay for the tail coverage. Many physicians will also tell you that the financial impact is no comparison to the psychological stress from being named in a lawsuit.

Case 8.20 Blaming the wrong person

A final example of frivolous lawsuits comes from Jennifer Silverman in *Family Practice News*.[24] A urologist was sued for a vasectomy failure after the patient's wife became pregnant. This occurred even though the patient's sperm count was checked at one week and one month. It was later discovered that the patient was not the father of the baby. This lawsuit was not only frivolous in the absence of medical negligence, but would also have been preventable had the patient consulted with his wife. The plaintiff attorney should also be faulted for using false information as the basis of his lawsuit.

Inherent errors of the practice

The practice of emergency medicine has inherent factors that make it prone to errors. A 2003 article in the *Annals of Emergency Medicine* commented on some of these errors in residency training. However, they also apply equally well to the emergency medicine attending. The article referred to the emergency department as an 'environment prone to error.'[25] 'Unique operating conditions of the ED environment include: the simultaneous management of several ill patients, a limited knowledge of patients' pre-existing medical conditions, high levels of diagnostic uncertainty, and high decision density.'[25] Additional obstacles are a 'loud and busy setting, where patients are often treated in crowded conditions with inadequate equipment. Care delivery is frequently interrupted, and there may be multiple transitions of care, often to staff who are fatigued or suffering circadian dysynchronicity resulting from insufficient recovery time from a shift change.'[25]

Patients who are seen in the emergency department are, by nature, going to have a greater percentage of adverse outcomes than patients who are seen in the office. This applies to whether the patients are admitted to the hospital or discharged home. The belief that admitted patients relieve the emergency physician of liability has now been shown to be a myth and should be abandoned. Traditionally, the role of the emergency physician was to stabilize a patient that needed hospitalization and then transfer care to the admitting physician. Emergency physicians frequently do not have the time or resources to unravel all of the medical problems that a patient may have on a particular visit. Despite this, ED doctors are more commonly involved in malpractice suits from admitted patients for failure to diagnose and for incomplete evaluations.

A common example would be the patient who presents with shortness of breath and has a chest X-ray that shows florid congestive heart failure. Although the patient is admitted and treated for heart failure, the shortness of breath does not improve and the patient is subsequently found to have a pulmonary embolus. The emergency physician is faulted for not discovering this in the emergency department. Emergency physicians are trained to get patients admitted as soon as admission criteria are met in order to maintain patient flow through a busy department and keep beds available. Unfortunately, whenever there is a delay in making a diagnosis or whenever the admitting physician fails to diagnose and an adverse outcome results, all treating physicians are named in the suit. This is becoming the standard of practice for plaintiff attorneys. The more physicians they can get named on the suit, the more likely they are to find someone at fault and the more money they are likely to obtain.

Since ED doctors cannot do much about changing their practice style due to the time and space constraints on their practice, there is little control that they have over this situation. Our advice is to remain vigilant for any possible diagnoses and state them to the admitting physician. Also, document this in the chart even if you do not work them up for it. This does not guarantee that you will be off the hook but it does help you formulate a defense should the need arise.

We have also discovered that many of the famous clichés are tailor-made for emergency medicine. Phrases like 'when it rains, it pours' and 'feast or famine' are accurate descriptors of our daily events. Unlike office practice settings where patients are given appointment times to maintain an orderly schedule, the emergency department waiting room has no maximum capacity. There may be times when the emergency physician will relax with an empty waiting room, and there will be times when 10 patients will come at one time with emergencies leaving the physician to hustle. During these hectic or 'rainy' times, the emergency physician does not have the option of yelling for 'mercy' or 'uncle' and ordering a hold on new patients. Instead, he may continue to see them 'pour' in. The ultimate example is the scene in New York City from September 11, 2001. Emergency physicians and nurses routinely stage mass casualty drills but not of the magnitude that the emergency physicians and nurses from New York experienced on that particular day.

The weight factor

America has an obesity problem and has an overweight society. Obesity is not only the basis of many medical problems; it also creates problems with the medical evaluation and treatment. It is much more difficult to perform procedures such as central line placement or lumbar puncture in larger people. Furthermore, the accuracy of some medical equipment is also limited by size such as gallbladder ultrasound or even X-rays. The major problem we see, however, is when you do not have available tests for a suspected disease because of a person's size.

A common example is the limit of most catheterization tables. At our facility, this is around 330 lbs. This certainly creates a problem because there are many people who are over this weight that have coronary artery disease. Besides the loss of diagnostic heart catheterization and/or percutaneous coronary intervention, many obese patients are poor candidates for the treadmill.

Case 8.21 Watching your weight

The second example is the evaluation for pulmonary embolism. We recently saw a patient who weighed 440 lbs for shortness of breath and pleuritic chest pain. He was a young 26-year-old male but had significant hypertension and an increased arterial-alveolar gradient on arterial blood gas with slight hypoxemia. We were the third of three different ED physicians to see this patient. All of the physicians had considered the diagnosis of pulmonary embolism but had no good diagnostic means to confirm it. We ordered cardiac tests, which were all negative. We also ordered an ultrasound of both legs, which were negative for deep venous thrombosis. He was too heavy for the tables that were used for CT pulmonary artery studies, ventilation-perfusion scans, and pulmonary arteriograms. Although we suspected that this man's hypoxia was due to obstructive sleep apnea and his pulmonary embolus risk was probably low, we did not want to continue to send this man home and have him return shortly thereafter. Therefore, we called the pulmonologist on call and recommended that the patient be admitted for evaluation and, if needed, instigation of treatment for sleep apnea and also an echocardiogram to evaluate for pulmonary hypertension. A pulmonary embolus might possibly be diagnosed with a transesophageal echocardiogram but the sensitivity for this test is low and his weight would probably limit the accuracy of the study.

Case 8.22 Weighing the options

Another dilemma with the obese patient comes when a lumbar puncture is needed. A colleague of ours saw a patient who weighed 415 lbs and presented to the ED with the 'worst headache of [his] life.' His head CT was negative for an intracranial bleed. The doctor wanted to proceed with a lumbar puncture but felt that it would be extremely difficult based on the patient's morbid size. The radiologist was ready to perform the procedure when it was discovered that the weight limit of the fluoroscopy table was 300 lbs. The patient, however, felt better after his CT scan, refused a lumbar puncture, and signed out against medical advice.

The increasing weight of American society is certainly a multi-faceted problem today. We must not only treat the medical complications of obesity, but we must also develop new technology to help us evaluate obese patients. Furthermore, clinicians must remember to use caution with these patients because their size may limit the sensitivity of your physical exam and clinical tests while precluding the use of other tests.

Case 8.23 The same problem again

Finally, we had an interesting case where the patient's size not only limited our diagnostic tests; it also affected his medical care. After an Arena League football game, a player weighing over 400 lbs was brought to our ED in full spinal immobilization. He had suffered a neck injury and was complaining of neck pain. Due to his broad shoulders, it was not possible to see his lower cervical and thoracic spine on X-rays. In addition, his weight was also beyond the capacity of the CT scanner in the hospital. Therefore, we had to arrange for him to go to an outpatient MRI facility. This task took several hours because the facility was not usually open on a Saturday night. After the patient was transported to the facility and had the scan, we received a report that it was 'negative.' During the return trip, however, the paramedics dropped the patient on his neck from the stretcher because he was too heavy. He was finally cleared hours later after another MRI.

Making judgment decisions that involve risks to the patient

There are times when the physician has to make a judgment decision whether to administer a medication or not. The medication may serve an immediate benefit to the patient's problem. Its administration, however, is also accompanied by possible complications. The physician must recommend (or decide in the event that the patient is incoherent without a durable power of attorney present) the choice that he feels is in the patient's best interest. On the other side of the coin, the physician must understand that the treatment may also cause serious and detrimental effects for the patient.

The classic example is the administration of fibrinolytics for patients with acute myocardial infarction or acute cerebrovascular accident. While the benefits of fibrinolytics substantially improve the morbidity and mortality of the acute event, the complication of bleeding can also lead to permanent injury or death. Similarly, the emergent treatment of status epilepticus sometimes leads to the administration of medications that may be detrimental. This usually occurs when the patient comes in status or is postictal and not able to give a history. The physician must try to stop the seizure without knowing what the patient is currently taking or the allergies that he or she may have.

Case 8.24 No time to wait for tests

A 42-year-old male was brought to our ED by the paramedics actively seizing for 15 minutes. He had a history of alcohol abuse and seizure disorder, and was currently taken Depakote and Dilantin. The paramedics noted that they were familiar with the patient and that he had a long history of non-compliance with his medications. He also had alcohol on his breath and was given 10 mg of valium without cessation of seizure activity. Blood sugar was within the normal range.

In the ED, he was given two doses of Ativan 2 mg intravenously without any effect on his seizure. He was also given thiamine and intravenous fluids for his alcohol abuse. Although his Dilantin level had not returned, we decided that it was time to give the patient Dilantin intravenously. We felt that his level would probably be low because of the paramedic's history and the frequent association of medicine non-compliance and alcoholism. In addition, in our ED Pyxis, there are only two types of intravenous medicines for seizures, Dilantin and benzodiazepines. Any other medication would have to be ordered and prepared from the pharmacy. Hence, the patient was loaded with Dilantin and his seizure activity stopped within five minutes.

He remained in a postictal state for the next two hours. During this time, his Dilantin level (drawn before the load) came back over two times the normal limit, while his Depakote level was subtherapeutic. We had iatrogenically worsened this patient's Dilantin toxicity. Given the circumstances, we had to make a judgment call to prevent this patient from hypoxic brain injury. Consequently, the seizure activity had ceased. The patient was treated for his toxicity and subsequently had a complete recovery.

The lack of equipment and/or facilities

We began this chapter talking about equipment failure. Uncontrollable errors may also result from lack of equipment or outdated equipment. Medical offices and hospitals spend a significant percentage of their budgets on medical supplies. Despite this large expenditure, we often cannot afford the equipment that we would like and sometimes run out of the equipment that we have. Inadequate equipment increases our medical liability in certain circumstances.

Case 8.25 A short supply

Our colleague, Bryce Tiller, MD, shared one of his cases with us. The case occurred while he was working in a small, rural emergency department during his residency. After a patient that he was treating for shortness of breath started to develop agonal breathing, he asked the nursing staff to get him a laryngoscope for oral intubation. The respiratory therapist informed him that the one laryngoscope the hospital had was being sterilized. Fortunately, the patient's breathing was stabilized with a non-rebreather mask until the local paramedics were able to bring him another laryngoscope.

This is only one of many examples that we could give for lack of equipment. There have been multiple occasions during our careers when we did not have the proper equipment to evaluate or treat a patient. Most instances are minor nuisances such as a lack of gonorrhea DNA probes or proper size vaginal speculums. Some, however, have been significant enough to make us want to pull our hair out. It is a physician's nightmare to not have a central line kit when a patient needs intravenous access or a lumbar puncture kit when meningitis is suspected. Although we have little control over the medical inventory, we should take it seriously when a nurse tells us that this 'is the last one.'

In a similar manner, lack of facilities also creates medical liability. Hospitals and clinics vary in the services and facilities that they offer. Medical conditions that require treatment that the facility cannot provide represent significant liabilities for the treating physician. The example that we are most familiar with is the treatment of pediatric patients. Our hospital, like many others, does not have pediatric inpatient facilities. Hospital marketing, however, encourages parents to bring their children to the emergency department regardless of the potential of disposition problems. In addition, the majority of these hospitals do not have pediatricians available for consultations. We saw an advertisement from a hospital that does not admit pediatric patients telling parents to 'bring your kids to our emergency department if you believe they may have meningitis.' The additional revenue from pediatric patients is nice for the hospitals if they are not offset by lawsuits that arise from not being able to treat, as illustrated in the following case.

Case 8.26 No friends to help

Selbst and Korin present a case, in *Preventing Malpractice Lawsuits in Pediatric Emergency Medicine*, where the circumstances above led to a hospital settlement.[26] An 11-month-old girl was seen at a clinic for fever, lethargy, and vomiting. Supportive care with Tylenol and a clear liquid diet was recommended without any diagnostic tests. When her condition did not improve, her parents called the clinic the following day and talked to a nurse. The nurse advised the parents against going to the ED and to continue supportive therapy. She did not discuss the conversation with the physician. Shortly later, the child was taken to an ED that did not have a pediatrician available. Although she was transferred to a facility with pediatricians six hours later, she died of meningitis. A settlement was made against the clinic and the initial ED for $170 000.

The medical clinic in this case obviously made a misdiagnosis and did not handle a callback very well. Hence, it is not surprising that they were included in the settlement. The authors did not, however, provide details of the child's care in the first emergency department. Assuming that the child had an advanced stage of meningitis when she presented to the ED and that everything was handled appropriately by the ED staff (antibiotics and hemodynamic support started immediately), the child's outcome would have probably been the same. Six hours is not too abnormal to get results

continued

from a lumbar puncture and arrange for a transfer (sometimes it takes 1–2 hours for the ambulance to come for transport). Given that these conditions were met, the first hospital was included in the settlement simply because the child was delayed in seeing a pediatrician.

Lawsuits concerning misrepresentation are becoming more popular in the medical malpractice field. The usual scenario occurs when the plaintiff claims that they assumed the physician they were seeing was board-certified or trained in the specific field of their problem. There are patients who come to the ED and believe that the physician that sees them is a specialist in the field that they need and do not realize that the ED physician will see them first. In the private offices, patients sometimes assume that resident physicians who are moonlighting are board-certified physicians. Hospitals, in this example, can also be charged for misrepresentation when they advertise for pediatric care and then fail to provide the inpatient services. In the presence of an adverse outcome, the plaintiff's argument will be that they were misled to believe that a pediatrician was available and that the unexpected delay resulted in the injury.

Problems with housestaff

We are all familiar with the hierarchy in medical academic institutions. The chain of command in progressively higher rank is: medical students, interns, senior residents, chief residents, and attending physicians. We discussed above that direct contact between the transferring and accepting physicians is required in patient transfers. This requirement will occasionally create confusion and consequently increased liability in certain situations.

As an attending physician, the transferring physician would ideally prefer to speak with the attending physician of the academic institution. In reality, however, most calls to medical academic centers are screened by the medical housestaff. The usual protocol is for the housestaff to discuss any possible transfers with their attending physicians. Therefore, direct contact between attending physicians is infrequently made. Housestaff physicians are not permitted by most hospitals to serve as 'accepting physicians' on transfer forms. What happens if an intern accepts a patient who is not authorized? How about when the housestaff makes a decision without consulting with their attending physician? The experience level of the housestaff member handling the phone call is extremely diverse and may adversely affect patient care decisions. One residency program had residents who were notoriously afraid about calling their attending physicians in the middle of the night. Therefore, potential patient transfers often had to wait until the morning hours. The following case highlights several of the potential problems in dealing with housestaff.

Case 8.27 Chain of command

An elderly man came to our emergency department after suffering a head injury. He was uncertain of what hit him on the head but believed that a tree branch had fallen on him. He had a massive headache but denied loss of consciousness or any neurologic symptoms. There were two moderate-size scalp lacerations with underlying hematomas on the top of his scalp.

Although his neurologic exam was normal, the questionable mechanism of injury and the moderate size of the injuries prompted us to order a CT scan of his head. Although there was no blood seen within the cranium, there was a significant amount of intracranial air seen along with a linear non-depressed skull fracture.

In the presence of an open skull fracture and its associated risks of intracranial infections and injuries, we felt that neurosurgical evaluation and/or admission was warranted. In addition, since the patient's history was extremely sketchy, we did not feel that he was a good candidate for discharge. However, our facility did not have neurosurgical coverage that night. Therefore, we called the local academic teaching hospital to discuss a patient transfer.

The housestaff physician that responded to our call was a surgery intern on the neurosurgery service. After hearing about the patient, he asked us what the significance of intracranial air meant and why the patient needed to be admitted. Our request to speak with the attending physician was denied as the intern stated that he would talk to his attending physician and call us back.

Fifteen minutes later, the intern called us back and said that his attending physician wanted us to send the patient home and follow up in the office. Again, we were denied the opportunity to speak with the attending physician. We asked for the name of the attending so that we could document the person giving this crucial recommendation. The intern gave us a name.

As we hesitantly prepared the patient for discharge, the intern called back. He now stated that his attending wanted us to transfer the patient to his hospital. We asked if the accepting physician was going to be the name that he gave us earlier. The intern replied that the name given earlier was that of his chief resident and that they had just spoken with their attending who overrode their previous orders.

This case illustrates the dilemmas that are inherent with any hierarchy, not just those of medicine. The subordinate members are responsible for screening and relieving their superiors of 'minor' or 'routine' tasks. The definitions of these tasks, however, are extremely broad, individual-dependent and subject to potential errors. Subordinate members may also be afraid of 'bothering' their superiors with 'trivial' problems to avoid being labeled as 'weak' and 'incompetent.' Furthermore, the experience level of the individual making critical decisions is often not optimal. Finally, in the case of dealing with housestaffs, the legal standard calls for direct contact between transferring and accepting physicians.

References

1 Guldner G and Leinen A (2003) Malpractice or misfortune? we, the jury, find the emergency physician... *EMpulse.* **8**(4): 23.
2 Simon RR and Brenner BE (1994) *Emergency Procedures and Techniques.* Williams & Wilkins, Baltimore, Maryland, 394.
3 Berek JS, Adashi EY and Hillard PA (1996) *Novak's Gynecology* (12e). Williams & Wilkins, Baltimore, Maryland, 263.
4 (2003) *Physicians Financial News.* **21**(12): 18.
5 Booth B (2003) Is this trip really necessary? *American Medical News.* **46**(34): 9.
6 Albert T (2003) Physician appeals award in lawsuit over waiting times. *American Medical News.* **46**(31): 1, 4.
7 Edwards FJ (2002) *The M & M Files: morbidity and mortality rounds in emergency medicine.* Hanley & Belfus, Inc., Philadelphia, Pennsylvania, 41–2.
8 Pennachio DL (2003) I didn't know I was suing you! *Medical Economics.* **80**(21): 80.
9 Connell EB (2004) The cost of frivolous lawsuits. *Family Practice News.* **34**(2): 14.
10 Albert T (2004) Lawyers try new tacks in malpractice suits. *American Medical News.* **47**(6): 21.
11 Starr DS (2004) What not to do when you leave a medical practice. *Cortlandt Forum.* **17**(4): 82–5.
12 Starr DS (2004) What not to do when you leave a medical practice. *Cortlandt Forum.* **17**(4): 85.
13 Starr DS (2004) A prompt referral doesn't protect this FP. *Cortlandt Forum.* **17**(1): 71–2.
14 Starr DS (2004) A prompt referral doesn't protect this FP. *Cortlandt Forum.* **17**(1): 72.
15 Horn C, Caldwell DH and Osborn DC (2000) *Law For Physicians: an overview of medical legal issues.* American Medical Association, Chicago, Illinois, 60.
16 Wear-Finkle DJ (2000) *Medicolegal Issues in Clinical Practice: a primer for the legally challenged.* Rapid Psychler Press, Port Huron, Michigan, 92.
17 Edwards FJ (2002) *The M & M Files: morbidity and mortality rounds in emergency medicine.* Hanley & Belfus, Inc., Philadelphia, Pennsylvania, 115.
18 Merry A and McCall Smith A (2001) *Errors, Medicine, and the Law.* Cambridge University Press, Cambridge, United Kingdom, 12–13.
19 Lowes R (2004) Frivolous suits, These doctors bite back. *Medical Economics.* **80**(18): 41–51.
20 Albert T (2004) Ob-gyn sues West Virginia trial lawyers. *American Medical News.* **47**(4): 2, 4.
21 Albert T (2004) Ob-gyn sues West Virginia trial lawyers. *American Medical News.* **47**(4): 4.
22 Albert T (2004) Panel documents frivolous lawsuits. *American Medical News.* **47**(7): 1, 4.
23 Albert T (2004) Panel documents frivolous lawsuits. *American Medical News.* **47**(7): 1.
24 Silverman J (2004) Physicians fight against 'frivolous' lawsuits. *Family Practice News.* **34**(10): 72.
25 Hevia A and Hobgood C (2003) Medical errors during residency: to tell or not to tell. *Annals of Emergency Medicine.* **42**(4): 565.
26 Selbst SM and Korin JB (1999) *Preventing Malpractice Lawsuits in Pediatric Emergency Medicine.* American College of Emergency Physicians, Dallas, Texas, 139.

Chapter 9

Other legal issues involving emergency physicians: part I

- Subpoenas
- Patient dumping issues
- Necessity of transfers
- When does a patient who is discharged need transfer papers?
- Reluctant attendings
- Blood-borne exposures
- Liability of patients who are held in the emergency department
- The emergency physician as social worker
- Suicidal patients
- Homicidal patients
- Patients that may require life-saving resuscitation
- Transportation
- Homeless patients
- Liability of consultants
- Which physician do we call for orders?

Emergency physicians evaluate and treat myriad patients from all aspects of life. We treat all patients regardless of situation or income. This includes criminals, sexual assault victims, crime victims, children of abuse, etc. When we treat these types of patient, we become involved with their subsequent legal issues. It would be hard to find an emergency physician who has practiced for any significant amount of time and has not been given a subpoena or has not appeared in court. However, we do not receive much education concerning these legal issues in our training. Therefore, this chapter is composed from a combination of our clinical experiences and our readings.

Subpoenas

Guidner and Leinen provide an extremely informative article concerning subpoenas for emergency physicians in *EMpulse*.[1] They explain that ED doctors are usually served a subpoena when they behave as witnesses for potential testimony in a court of law. A typical example would be a physician who treats an assault victim. The physician is then asked to testify in a case in which the assailant is tried. 'A subpoena is served on a witness, not a defendant.'[2]

To better illustrate the role of a witness in a subpoena, the above authors define the two types of witnesses. Most physicians are familiar with the expert witness in malpractice lawsuits. 'An expert witness is someone hired by those involved in a case to provide an opinion (in retrospect) regarding various aspects of the case.'[2] Their role in the case is strictly voluntary. In contrast, the other type of witness, the percipient witness, does not always have the choice to participate in a case. This witness has personal knowledge about the events of the case. Emergency physicians most commonly find themselves serving as this latter type of witness due to the nature of their work. Furthermore, the cases where we are most likely to be summoned are the ones that involve criminal activities. However, we may occasionally treat patients that are later involved in civil lawsuits. Guidner and Leinen give the example of the patient that is treated for injuries sustained after a ladder collapses.[2] The treating ED physician may later get a subpoena for a lawsuit involving the manufacturer of the defective ladder.

Most states mandate that a subpoena be served in person to the recipient. However, in most jurisdictions, individuals may elect a proxy who is able to accept a subpoena on their behalf. In our practice, we have noticed that the courts make a few notable attempts to contact us in person. However, due to our shift schedule, it is sometimes difficult to get in touch with us during the days that we are not working. Therefore, it has become common practice for subpoenas to be left in our mailboxes and not delivered in person. We would add that we have never designated a proxy to accept subpoenas for us in our practice. This raises the question whether these indirectly issued subpoenas hold any legal merit. We do not have a concrete answer to this question.

Subpoenas can bring frustration for the emergency physician in many ways. They frequently do not list the name of the patient that the physician treated, making it impossible for the physician to pull any records for review. An example is an attempted murder case that we received a subpoena for two years ago. The case on the subpoena was titled 'The State of Florida versus John Doe.' We did not know anything about the case that the subpoena entailed until we arrived in the courtroom and discovered that our patient was the victim of John Doe.

During one summer in our practice, we received approximately 10 subpoenas in three months. All requested that we be available on certain dates (sometimes one subpoena will list several consecutive days for trial). These dates made it impossible for us to leave town for two consecutive months. As it turned out, all of these court dates were subsequently cancelled. Some subpoenas may request that you travel a substantial distance, thus creating another inconvenience. State laws vary on this issue so check with your hospital attorney.

Occasionally, your subpoena will be on a day that you were scheduled to work. Not only do you have to find coverage for your shift, you will likely receive minimal or no compensation for your lost wages. We were unaware of how witnesses were compensated when we attended the 'The State of Florida versus John Doe' case above. The attorneys involved never discussed that we were entitled to any compensation. We went to the trial and were not only questioned on the facts of the case but were also repeatedly asked for our medical opinions. We served our duty and did not realize until later that we were entitled to a minimal stipend. Guidner and Leinen give an example of a percipient witness in California receiving $35 a day plus twenty cents per mile of travel.[3] This minuscule stipend would not excite most physicians (or anyone else for that matter). However, Guidner and Leinen recommend that physicians should request to be paid in a similar fashion as expert witnesses if their medical expertise is inquired about in addition to the facts of the case.

We were subpoenaed and testified for the state attorney in a sexual assault case a few months ago. The subpoenae was served two working days prior to our scheduled shift in a city four hours away. We explained that it was impossible for us to attend this trial and be at our scheduled shift. We would also endure a significant loss of income. The explanation was to no avail to the state attorney. We had to call the attorney's office five times and talk to four different people before someone finally revealed that we were indeed entitled to compensation that was set by the county for physician testimony. The take-home message is to know your legal rights. The experience, however, of being in the courtroom and testifying is priceless because it enables one to experience how distressing it is to be on trial. We encourage all physicians to get as much of this experience as possible but remember to get compensated for it.

Good news, though, is that most subpoenas are not set in stone. The majority of subpoenas that we have received have been cancelled. Furthermore, since the physician is not usually the defendant in a subpoena, most attorneys are willing to accommodate any scheduling conflicts that the physician may have and assist them with any questions. We have also experienced that judges are fairly lenient if the physician has a legitimate problem with the subpoena.

The other type of subpoena that is often given to physicians is a subpoena for medical records. These requests often involve worker's compensation cases, nursing home cases, etc. Physicians must be careful with these situations because they may get themselves in legal difficulties if the records are released without proper authorization. This usually means that the subpoena is accompanied by either a judge's signature or a patient's consent. The attorney's signature and order, by themselves, do not allow the physician to release a patient's records.

The last remark about subpoenas is to not ignore them. Most of our colleagues in the emergency department proudly boast that they simply slip subpoenas into the trash bucket and have never received any repercussions. 'Once the first subpoena is ignored, the attorney will issue a second, along with a copy to the judge. If the physician ignores the second subpoena, he or she is subjected to fine and jail time (although jail time is unlikely). Additionally, should the physician's failure to appear result in monetary damages to either party, the physician owes that party $500 plus all damages.'[3]

Patient dumping issues

The information in this section is extracted from *A Pocket Guide: legal issues impacting emergency medicine*.[4] Congress enacted The Emergency Medical Treatment and Active Labor Act to prevent hospitals from refusing to treat indigent patients. Under this law, any patient who presents to an emergency department requesting an examination is entitled to one regardless of the patient's ability to pay. It is mandatory for the hospital to provide the medical screening evaluation to determine if an emergent condition exists. Furthermore, this exam must be performed before the assessment of the patient's financial status.

Emergency conditions are defined as any condition that, without immediate medical attention, would result in any or all of the following:[4]

1 jeopardizing the health of an individual (including an unborn child)
2 causing serious impairment to bodily functions
3 causing serious dysfunction of any bodily organ or part and
4 (for the pregnant patient having contractions) insufficient time for the safe transfer to another facility before delivery, or, that the transfer may pose a threat to the health or safety of the woman or the unborn child.

Once it is determined that an emergent condition exists, the hospital is required to stabilize the patient by either:[4]

1 conducting further medical examinations and treatments in order to stabilize the condition or
2 transferring the individual to another facility in compliance with other rules regarding transfer.

Note that there are conditions that must be met before a patient can be transferred.[4] The physician must determine that the transfer is medically necessary. The patient must give informed consent for the transfer. Informed consent means that the indications, risks, and benefits of the transfer are explained to the patient. The receiving facility must have the ability to care for the patient. Finally, the transferring facility must make reasonable arrangements for transportation.

Many clinicians will believe that it is foolish to not comply with the above rules and endure the hefty penalties (financially and professionally). In actual clinical practice, however, the scenarios are not always black and white and are sometimes left in a gray zone.

Case 9.1 On your property

For example, the emergency medical services bring a patient to your emergency department. They are then physically on your premises with a patient that is requesting an examination. The paramedics then discover that they traveled to the wrong hospital and your triage nurse tells them the direction to the correct facility. The paramedics transport the patient to the other facility without a screening examination from your facility. This is not an uncommon scenario in emergency practice. It is also a violation of the EMTALA laws because the patient did not receive a screening examination to determine if an emergent condition existed that may require stabilization. The receiving facility is required by law to report the facility that did not perform the screening examination. This requirement is independent of whether the patient has an adverse outcome from the transfer.

Case 9.2 Stretching the definition of emergency

The second example is of a patient who presented to the emergency department with abdominal pain and the evaluation revealed that he had acute appendicitis. The surgeon on call was asked to see the patient. After he

continued

inquired about the duration of the abdominal pain and whether a perforation was present on the CT scan, he informed the emergency physician that the patient was stable enough to have the surgery a few hours from the time of the phone consultation. He noted that the patient was on a particular health plan in which he did not participate. He also stated that the surgeons at the other hospital treated patients on that health plan. He felt that the patient was stable enough for transfer and requested that the patient be transferred to the other hospital. Is this a case of patient dumping and of EMTALA violation? Strong arguments could be made for both sides. These preceding cases are only two scenarios where unintentional violations in the EMTALA laws can be made along with their accompanying severe consequences.

Case 9.3 May I see your ID?

The third case is similar to the second with a little twist. A 16-year-old who was six feet tall and weighed 250 lbs presented to the emergency department of a hospital that did not have pediatricians and pediatric subspecialists. He complained of lower abdominal pain and was found to have a ruptured appendix on a CT scan. He was comfortably medicated and his vitals were stable. The surgeon on call stated that the hospital did not treat children and asked the emergency physician to transfer the child to a hospital that did treat children.

When the ED physician contacted the surgeon from the other hospital, the surgeon stated that the child was 'equivalent to an adult' and should be treated by the initial on-call surgeon. He felt that a transfer of this patient would be an EMTALA violation. The ED physician called his surgeon again and requested that the surgeon evaluate the patient. The first surgeon came and evaluated the patient. He then called the surgeon from the other facility. He offered to take care of the child at his facility but stated that he would file an EMTALA violation against the second surgeon for not accepting the child to a hospital that had medical facilities (pediatric ward with pediatricians) that his hospital did not have. He offered the example of a similar-aged child who developed an arrhythmia after surgery and was unable to get a cardiology consultation because none of the staff cardiologists would see a pediatric patient (regardless of size or weight). After further consideration, the surgeon from the second facility accepted the child. We have seen similar cases where EMTALA violations were filed from both sides.

Case 9.4 We are not having a baby

A 20-year-old primigravida female with a 31-week intrauterine pregnancy presented to the emergency department complaining of lower abdominal pain. The hospital policy was to have all patients with pregnancies that are

continued

over 20 weeks and a possible pregnancy-related complaint sent to Labor and Delivery for initial evaluation and then to the ED if necessary. Therefore, the admitting clerk called the labor and delivery nurse and informed her that there was a patient to evaluate.

The nurse spoke with the patient on the phone and informed her repeatedly that her obstetrician did not practice at this hospital and that she could not be seen here. Fortunately, another nurse overheard this potential EMTALA violation and intercepted the conversation before the patient was sent off to another hospital. When she was evaluated in Labor and Delivery, she was found to be 9 cm dilated and completely effaced with active contractions every two minutes and a bulging bag of membranes.

Although this patient's active labor was discovered and treated without any complications, this case could have easily resulted in an unfavorable outcome for all parties involved. The patient could have delivered her baby in transit to another hospital with hemodynamic and cardiovascular complications to her and/or her baby. The hospital would have been found in violation of the EMTALA laws and would have been subjected to a huge fine and loss of financial support. Finally, the hospital employee responsible for the violation would likely lose his or her job and have problems with finding a similar job in the future because of this huge error.

The last caveat regarding transfer is that all patients should be stabilized as much as possible before transfer. Stabilization measures must take into consideration potential problems that may arise during transfer. Typical examples would include intubating a patient who may lose his or her airway and placing a chest tube for a patient with a pneumothorax. There are situations, however, where stabilization measures may vary with the treating physician. Because the sending physician can be found guilty of an EMTALA violation if the receiving physician does not feel that proper stabilization is performed, the sending physician should always discuss the appropriate stabilization measures with the accepting physician before transferring the patient.

Case 9.5 Tune them up first

Edwards presents a case, in *The M & M Files*, where an EMTALA violation was filed for inappropriate patient stabilization.[5] While cutting trees, a 75-year-old man was struck on the head with a branch. The man lost consciousness and was taken to a small ED by his nephew. He was initially found to be confused and agitated with a large scalp laceration. A hard neck collar was placed in triage, but the patient refused to leave it in place.

After the ED physician examined the patient, he decided that the best immediate action was to transfer the patient by helicopter to the nearest trauma center. He did not feel that a CT scan would alter the treatment at his facility. Twenty minutes later, when the helicopter arrived, the patient became unconscious and started to posture. The physician notified the

continued

trauma center of these findings and administered mannitol per its request. Shortly later, during the flight, the patient vomited and went into respiratory distress. The patient became pulseless and apneic and subsequent intubation and resuscitation attempts were unsuccessful. A large subdural hematoma with brain herniation was discovered during the autopsy.

An EMTALA violation was filed by the trauma center against the smaller hospital for inadequate stabilization of the patient before transfer. They contended that the patient's airway was not protected and his neck was not evaluated before the transfer. The smaller hospital and its ED physician were both given fines despite their appeals. In this case, the ED physician correctly did not waste time with a CT scan at his facility. He also arranged for the patient to receive neurosurgical intervention as rapidly as possible. He did not, however, anticipate the likelihood of the patient losing his airway from a large neurologic insult and the difficulty of intubation in transit. Furthermore, although it is debatable whether the patient needed further stabilization of his neck, the ED physician would have helped his case by asking the trauma center about its specific stabilization requirements.

Necessity of transfers

We have seen many requests to transfer patients during our career in emergency medicine. The numerous managed care organizations (MCO) and medical reimbursements of our medical system frequently lead to requests of transfers for non-medical reasons. MCOs sometimes deny authorization of medical treatment at other facilities and want their patients sent to their own facilities. In addition, patients that receive care at a Veterans Administration Hospital frequently ask to be sent to a government facility for hospitalization.

We discussed in Chapter 7 the dangers of patient transfers. Even in the event of a transfer that is medically necessary, things may go wrong that the physician may be faulted for (i.e. decompensation while en route, incomplete records sent, etc.). Can one imagine how disastrous it would be for the physician if these unfortunate events occurred in a transfer that was not medically necessary? Furthermore, do not let a denial of authorization and request for transfer distract you from your commitment to stabilize the patient.

Case 9.6 Getting the runaround

Selbst and Korin, in *Preventing Malpractice Lawsuits in Pediatric Emergency Medicine*, present such a case.[6] After an 18-month-old child was brought to the ED for wheezing, lethargy, vomiting, and diarrhea, her vital signs were notably abnormal and were as follows: pulse 130 beats/minute, respirations 40 breaths/minute, and temperature of 106.6°F. Despite these findings, she was transferred to the pediatric acute care clinic in the hospital.

In the clinic, the child was treated for difficulty breathing and a seizure.

continued

Afterwards, the staff contacted the MCO physician, who requested that the child be transferred to an affiliated hospital and that no blood tests be performed. The child went into cardiac arrest approximately 20 minutes after arriving at the receiving hospital and died. The cause of death upon autopsy was Streptococcus pneumoniae sepsis, which was worsened by the child's congenital asplenia.

A lawsuit was filed against the physicians involved and the two hospitals. It was not hard to see why the family was awarded $1.3 million in this case. The first hospital did not evaluate and stabilize an unstable patient before transfer. In addition, the patient was inappropriately triaged to a step-down unit from the ED where she subsequently had respiratory and neurological complications. In essence, the initial hospital violated the EMTALA laws in transferring this patient and could face federal penalties. Could this hospital defend that this transfer was of medical necessity?

The second facility and the MCO would also have a difficult time defending the events of this case. The MCO made serious errors in not authorizing emergent treatment for this child and for recommending an ill-advised transfer for the child. Its affiliated hospital, likewise, made an error by accepting this patient without prior medical stabilization. Therefore, adverse outcomes can become difficult or impossible to defend when we allow the politics of medicine to be the driving force for our treatment.

Case 9.7 You came to the wrong place

We were faced with similar circumstances during one case in our ED. We received a call from the emergency medical services that they were bringing in an 18-month-old with a first time seizure and a fever. Since we are not a pediatric hospital, we asked the paramedics to inform the child's mother of this and the necessity of transfer if hospitalization were required. The paramedics refused to do so.

Upon arrival to the ED, the child appeared postictal and had a temperature of 99.5°F. When we told the child's mother that the child may need to be transferred for hospitalization because this did not appear to be a typical case of a febrile seizure, she became upset that the paramedics has not told her this. She requested that the child be transferred immediately to a pediatric hospital. The patient's pediatrician also requested this when we contacted him. We did not feel that this request was appropriate at the time because the child needed an evaluation to determine stability. The etiology of the seizure was still unknown and the child had the potential to have another one during transportation.

Hence, we proceeded to order a head CT, blood work, a urinalysis, and a chest X-ray. The tests were all unremarkable with the exception of a quarter-size foreign body in the child's esophagus. After discussing the case with the on-call otolaryngologist, it was determined that the benefit of transferring the child to a pediatric facility for treatment outweighed the risk of transfer. Therefore, the child was transferred at this time.

When does a patient who is discharged need transfer papers?

Regardless of how long you have been practicing emergency medicine, this question is never answered with certainty. It is one of the most frequently discussed topics of emergency departmental meetings. Transfers are not always as black and white as they sound. Is a nursing home patient returning to a nursing home considered a transfer? Is a patient treated in the emergency department and going to an alcohol rehabilitation facility considered a transfer? How about the patient that the ED physician wants to admit but the admitting physician wants to see in her office first? A situation that was common in an ED where we used to practice was when the CT scanner would malfunction. During these times, we would send patients to another hospital to get their CT scan but not receive any treatment there. Since they were returning to us for treatment, did they represent transfers? These are all not clear-cut cases of patient transfer.

Case 9.8 Did you see what I saw?

A 21-year-old man was brought to our facility by ambulance. He had suffered multiple bites to his face by his dog. Although the man had a history of depression, and alcohol and drug abuse, he appeared totally coherent and was not actively homicidal or suicidal. He had been drinking but his alcohol level was less than the state legal limit. His wounds were very superficial and were cleaned and dressed.

Shortly after his arrival, a local police officer arrived in the emergency department. She stated that she was just at his house. The people there 'were partying and using drugs.' She did not feel that it was safe for him to return to it and she felt that he should be a Marchment Act. We were not sure why the patient should be a Marchment Act and told her that the patient did not give us any reason in the emergency department to warrant it. Furthermore, the patient had told her that he was willing to go for psychiatric treatment. She filled out the police form of the Marchment Act and took him to another hospital after our evaluation was completed. This is because our hospital did not have psychiatrists.

We felt that we did not have anything to do with the Marchment Act because it was completed by the police officer. The officer signed the forms based on events that occurred outside of the hospital. We treated and discharged this patient in the same manner as that of any other patient. However, when the officer took the patient to the other hospital, the administrator at the other facility called to inform us that we had performed an improper transfer and threatened to report it as an EMTALA violation. We informed her that we had not transferred the patient. We felt that our treatment of the patient and the police officer's decision to Marchment Act the patient and transfer him to a psychiatric facility were two separate entities. We felt that the EMTALA guidelines were met.

We realize that the correct interpretation of this case is debatable. The

continued

other hospital brought the issue to our risk management but decided to 'let it slide' and did not report it. In other words, they did not know the answer either. The simplest way to stay out of trouble with regard to transfer papers is to remember the dictum, 'if in doubt, fill them out.'

Reluctant attendings

Every ED physician can list one or two attending physicians on his hospital's medical staff who are always unwilling to admit a patient. These individuals are 'iron walls' and will not let an admission penetrate into their medical service. They frequently return the ED's call with great annoyance. They will also tend to admit only the patients who are having obvious serious medical conditions (e.g. hypoxia, hyperkalemia, myocardial infarction, etc.). Patients who have uncertain diagnoses (e.g. abdominal pain with a tender abdomen and normal labs, chest pain with cardiac risk factors and normal labs, pneumonia with history of chronic obstructive disease but no hypoxia) are often not acceptable admissions for these physicians. We are fortunate that these reluctant physicians are the exception and not the norm. The majority of the physicians that we work with share the same goal of thorough, quality medical care that is consistent with the standard of care.

These situations can be difficult and stressful for the ED physician to handle and may lead him to make a decision that is not in the patient's best interest. ED physicians have limited equipment, history, and time with which to evaluate patients. Therefore, the etiology of the symptoms may not always be evident after the evaluation. However, there will often still be emergent conditions that have not fully manifested. Therefore, refusing to admit a patient just because a definite diagnosis was not evident on the ED evaluation is a dangerous practice.

Most malpractice errors in emergency medicine occur when ED physicians discharge patients with a severe evolving disease process or a disease process that is occult at the time of the evaluation. Emergency physicians learn from these adverse outcomes. They also learn from the patients who return unimproved and are subsequently found to have a severe medical condition. Therefore, whenever an emergency physician feels that a patient should be admitted, it is often because he or she has experienced similar scenarios, which have resulted in unfavorable outcomes when the patients were not admitted. In addition, the ED physician may have an uneasy feeling about sending the patient home (e.g. because the patient does not have a good support system or is unable to follow instructions) and can only be reassured through direct communication and observation of the patient.

The emergency department is sometimes the 'last stop' in the medical evaluation. Patients will go to their primary care physician for a medical condition and receive treatment. If there is no improvement in this treatment, they will either return to their physician or go to the emergency department. Patients are aware that the emergency department is equipped with an abundance of medical technology and medical specialists. Consequently, if a patient is discharged from an emergency department, they are often under the impression that nothing further can be done for them. This impression may make them more hesitant to seek further medical care. This is in stark contrast to the patient treated by their primary physician who is often told to go to the emergency department if they are not better. Therefore, by the inherent nature of this process, there will be a significant number of patients with uncertain diagnoses that ED physicians must admit to the hospital.

Case 9.9 Every patient looks great from your home

Edwards presents a case, in *The M & M Files*, of a 46-year-old man who came to the ED with nausea, vomiting, and black stools for one day.[7] He had a prior history of a gastrointestinal bleed but had stable vital signs and a normal physical examination with the exception of dark-colored stool that was hemoccult-positive on rectal exam. His nausea had resolved with intravenous fluids and his blood tests and X-rays were unremarkable. He had one further melanotic stool in the ED so his primary care physician was contacted concerning admission.

The primary physician 'chided the emergency physician for wanting to admit a stable patient who could just as easily be evaluated on an outpatient basis.'[7] He requested that the patient receive more fluids and be discharged so that he could be re-evaluated in the morning. The ED physician agreed reluctantly to this plan.

After returning home, the patient continued to have melanotic stools and eventually had a syncopal episode. He returned to the ED and was admitted. An endoscopy showed an actively bleeding duodenal ulcer. The primary physician was unsupportive of the ED physician when he stated that he would not have discharged the patient had he 'known how sick the patient looked.'[7] This dilemma can be prevented by good communication between the ED physician and the consultant. The consultant should also maintain a low threshold to evaluate a patient in the ED if they are uncertain of the patient's clinical status.

So how do we recommend handling difficult situations like this? The first and easiest step is to try to convince the attending physician to admit the patient if you feel that the patient should not go home. A good, experienced clinician is usually right with his intuition and should stand behind it unless he is over-whelmingly convinced otherwise by the attending physician. As emergency physicians, we generally have a good feel of the patients that need to be admitted. Edwards states that 'when a disagreement about patient disposition arises, the emergency physician retains the right to request (i.e. demand) that the admitting physician come and personally evaluate a patient that the emergency physician feels should be admitted.'[8] In the event that the attending physician refuses to see the patient, the conflict should be brought to the attention of the consultant physician's department chief. If you still do not have an admitting physician at this point, you have one of two options. You can either find some-one else to admit the patient (i.e. another internist or a specialist) or you can observe the patient in the emergency department. Although the hospital staff and administration discourages the latter because it consumes hospital labor and space, it may be in the best interest of the patient.

One final point to emphasize on this subject: we encourage all emergency physicians to stand their ground on any patient that they feel strongly should be admitted. However, your goal is not to win every battle with a reluctant attending. After all, no one is correct 100% of the time and these reluctant attendings are also our colleagues and often our friends. You must know which battles to fight and which to concede.

Blood-borne exposures

Emergency physicians commonly evaluate patients after blood and body fluid exposures. Although there are a number of diseases that can be transmitted by blood and other body fluids, we will limit this discussion to the most concerning one, human immunodeficiency virus (HIV). Exposure can be categorized as occupational and non-occupational. Non-occupational exposure can further be divided into: unprotected intercourse, illicit drug use, and sexual assault. McCausland et al. did a study published in the Annals of Emergency Medicine concerning HIV post-exposure prophylaxis in non-occupational exposure.[9]

This study surveyed emergency physicians and found that they routinely offered HIV post-exposure prophylaxis to patients with occupational exposure. However, the study also showed that prophylaxis was offered less frequently to patients after sexual assault and even less frequently to patients with unsafe sexual practices or patients with injection drug use.[9] 'This stratification of offering HIV post-exposure prophylaxis is inversely proportional to the numbers of new infections caused by exposure type in the United States ... The vast majority of new HIV infections in the United States occur after unprotected sex and illicit drug use, whereas a small percentage of new infections are believed to be after sexual assault and occupational exposure.'[9]

The article from the Annals of Emergency Medicine also emphasizes that the Center for Disease Control and Prevention (CDC) 'neither recommends for or against offering HIV post-exposure prophylaxis after unsafe sexual practices or injection drug use exposure or after sexual assault.'[10] However, certain states have developed specific guidelines for handling some of the non-occupational situations. This is partly because there have been no studies confirming the efficacy of prophylaxis in non-occupational exposure. However, there have been documented studies confirming the benefits of prophylaxis in occupational exposure and the results from these studies could probably be extrapolated to the cases of non-occupational exposure. With this in mind and the potential legal implications of not offering HIV prophylaxis, we recommend that all blood and body fluids exposure be given equal consideration for HIV prophylaxis. This does not mean that we place every exposure on prophylaxis. Each individual case needs to be assessed on the risk profile of disease transmission. 'This risk profile takes into consideration the type of exposure, the likelihood that the source patient is HIV positive, and the amount of time after exposure.'[10] We also encourage hospitals to develop protocols for prophylaxis of non-occupational exposures in the same manner that most have for occupational exposures.

Liability of patients who are held in the emergency department

Most emergency departments are overfilled not only from patient overcrowding, but also from admitted patients that remain in the department due to unavailability of beds or nurses. The latter is becoming a more common problem with the current state of nursing shortage. At many hospitals, patients are kept in the emergency department not because there are no beds available but because there is no one to take care of the patient on the medical ward.

While these patients remain in the emergency department, they remain the responsibility of the emergency attending. Any medical complication that accompanies the patient while in the department can become a legal liability for the ED physician. Two excellent examples are the development of pressure ulcers and the development of deep venous thrombosis.

It is commonly written in the medical literature that a pressure ulcer can develop as early as two hours after immobilization of a vulnerable area. Patients that are admitted tend to be immobile, have poor nutritional status, and have chronic medical conditions. All of these factors, along with the inexperience of some emergency physicians and nurses at treating (or preventing) pressure ulcers, contribute to the likelihood of pressure ulcer development in the emergency department. In patients with established pressure ulcers, the emergency physician may be legally faulted if the ulcer becomes worse. Therefore, consider prophylactic measures to prevent ulcers from developing (e.g. change the patient's position), treat existing ulcers (e.g. avoid further pressure on the ulcer, debride necrotic tissue from the ulcer), and document existing ulcers (e.g. photography).

Deep venous thrombosis (DVT) is another condition that could potentially develop in the hospitalized patient. For the same reasons as those in the preceding paragraph, these patients are also at risk for developing DVTs. Similarly, emergency physicians are not routinely concerned with DVT prophylaxis. This is because most patients do not stay in the ED long enough to develop a blood clot. A few years ago, admitting physicians were shown at our hospital to underuse prophylaxis for DVTs. Therefore, our hospital developed a protocol where they automatically place a DVT prophylaxis protocol into every admitted patient's chart to remind the physician. The emergency physician, unfortunately, does not receive this reminder and is usually not aware of how long the patient is going to wait in the department when admission orders are given. Our proposed solution is to have the same hospital protocol extend to the emergency department for every admitted patient. Deep venous thrombosis and its complications are increasing in incidence. Concurrently, malpractice suits involving DVTs are also increasing.

Consultants often evaluate patients in the emergency department and write orders for the patient. Every (or almost every) emergency physician will probably admit that they have been guilty of assuming that the consultant who has seen and written orders for a patient in the ED has taken complete responsibility for the patient. Each of us can also remember cases where this assumption is not true and we learned the hard way that our responsibility to the patient does not end until the patient is physically out of the department.

Case 9.10 Who is the boss?

Edwards presents a case, in *The M & M Files,* where an assumption by an ED physician led to his criticism.[11] A 77-year-old man with a history of diverticulosis and diabetes came to the ED with several days of nausea, vomiting, diarrhea, and abdominal pain. He had a temperature of 100.8°F, pulse of 120 beats/minute, and a blood pressure of 105/59 mm Hg. He appeared dehydrated and toxic and had decreased breath sounds with left lower quadrant tenderness, guarding, and rebound. His abdominal X-ray showed an ileus and free air under the diaphragm.

The ED physician's impression was acute peritonitis from a ruptured diverticulum and immediately contacted the surgeon even before all of the tests had returned. Although the surgeon promptly saw the patient and ordered intravenous antibiotics for him, he did not order any intravenous fluids. The patient was finally taken to the surgical suite 3½ hours later but the surgery was delayed another two hours because the anesthesiologist felt that the patient was not adequately hydrated. The patient did well with his surgery but the ED physician still received a complaint from the anesthesiologist for not hydrating the patient.

This scenario is not infrequent in the emergency setting. As emergency physicians, we would like to sign off patients as soon as we can obtain another physician to assume their care. This enables us to address other patients who may be more critical or have not been seen by a physician. We agree with the anesthesiologist's frustration that the patient should have received better care in the emergency department. Certainly, any patient that remains in the department is the responsibility of the ED physician. The surgeon, however, should also share a portion of the blame in this case. He assumed care and prepared the patient for surgery but did not plan to hydrate the patient. Some surgeons are particular about the medications that are given to their patients preoperatively. Furthermore, is it expected of the emergency physician to review every admission order to discover what needs to be added? Therefore, although we encourage ED physicians to be aware of the treatment of admitted patients in the ED, we feel that the admitting physician should accept some culpability in this case.

The emergency physician as social worker

As we discussed previously, emergency physicians see and treat diverse groups of patients. Patients will present to the emergency department with medical, mental, and social problems. We have addressed the medical and mental problems in the previous chapters. Some patients, however, will come to the ED or are brought to the ED by their families because they cannot take care of themselves at home or their families cannot manage them at home any longer. This is not uncommon. Most EDs have social workers during business hours to address this problem. However, during evening and night time hours, the ED physician also serves as the social worker and must arrange the disposition for these patients.

These patients usually have stable medical processes without acute exacerbations and do not meet any standard medical admission criteria. However, they or their family would like them to be admitted. This common dilemma leaves the ED physician in a 'Catch 22.' If he is adamant that admission is not required, he automatically becomes the 'bad doctor.' This could result in complaints to hospital administration, state health agencies, and unfavorable comments concerning the ED physician to their private physician. Also, if the patient returns home and suffers an injury because there was no one to care for them (e.g. falls from unassisted walking), the ED physician may be legally blamed for not honoring the patient or the family's request.

On the other hand, if the ED physician insists to the primary physician she needs to admit a patient because of social and not medical reasons, the primary physician may eventually lose faith in the ED physician. A difficult situation is when the patient does not have a primary physician and they want to be admitted. Attempting to convince the on-call physician of this situation is usually a futile effort. Our best advice for these situations is to tell the patient that you will exhaust every effort you can to admit them but there are no guarantees. Make sure they understand that you do not have the power to admit and that they understand all of the efforts that were made. We have found that even unsuccessful attempts are met with patient and family satisfaction in the presence of sincere efforts.

Case 9.11 Treating the hidden patient

Edwards writes about a case, in *The M & M Files*, where a patient's wife requested that her husband be admitted and became outraged when he was not.[12] The patient was a 69-year-old male with end-stage chronic obstructive pulmonary disease who came to the ED by ambulance with shortness of breath. He had been in the ED recently for the same problem and was seen by the social worker on that visit in an attempt to arrange for hospice care. After appropriate treatment and evaluation by the ED physician, the patient stated that his breathing had returned to baseline. The ED physician discussed the case with the patient's primary physician and they agreed to discharge the patient to home. The patient's wife was surprised with this decision and became hostile when the ED physician offered to call social services the following day to facilitate the enrollment into a hospice.

The patient was admitted the following day by his primary care physician after this physician had received repeated calls from the patient's wife. The wife and her two children filed separate complaints to the hospital administrator concerning the 'rude behavior of the emergency physician.' These complaints were placed in the physician's peer review file and the case was presented in morbidity and mortality rounds.

Although the ED physician carried out appropriate medical treatment and disposition protocols, he could have performed certain actions that might have prevented the complaint. Edwards makes an outstanding point by stating that 'the emergency physician failed to recognize that he was

continued

treating two patients – the husband and the wife.'[13] Furthermore, he adds 'nothing prevented the emergency physician from calling the primary doctor back and putting him on the phone with the wife to discuss options.'[14] We would add that the emergency physician could have emphasized to the wife that he would utilize every option available (e.g. calling the primary physician, calling the pulmonologist) but that he could not make any guarantees because of the lack of the power to act as an admitting physician.

Another common example where the ED physician has to serve as a social worker is in the patient with a history of alcohol abuse who presents requesting admission for detoxification. These patients are usually not actively withdrawing from alcohol and do not meet medical criteria for admission. Furthermore, many physicians on the ED call roster will not admit an unassigned patient for alcohol detoxification. Unfortunately, these patients often are uninsured and do not have primary physicians. Consequently, the ED physician should call the community detoxification centers to seek placement for the patient. These attempts, however, are often unsuccessful due to the limited number of openings or the patient's lack of finances. Again, as in the previous example, you do your best for the patient and if you are unsuccessful, you explain to them your efforts and your limitations. In this case, we give them the number for the detoxification center and tell them to keep calling for the first available bed and give them the name of the substance abuse physician specialist in the community.

Another common example is the patient who treats the hospital like a motel. These patients would like to check in for a few days while they 'work out their social problems at home.' Because there are no good medical criteria to admit these patients, the emergency physician must act as a social worker in these scenarios.

Case 9.12 Stay and work out your problems

A case in point involves a 50-year-old female who presented to the emergency department with chest pain. Her only cardiac risk factor was hypertension and the area of pain on her chest was reproducible when we placed the stethoscope on her chest. Her cardiac work-up (EKG, cardiac enzymes, chest X-ray) was unremarkable. We felt that her pain was very atypical for coronary artery disease but she stated that she had to be admitted. When we asked her why, she answered, 'because I have a sick aunt at home and I don't want to have to take care of her.'

This answer did not strike us as a legitimate concern for her cardiac status. Instead, it made us feel like she expected us to help her take care of the social problems she had at home. Nevertheless, we called the cardiologist and expressed her concerns (and those of her family). He was also not impressed with her cardiac story but instructed us to send her over to his

continued

office (which was actually next door to the hospital) for a stress test. This gesture should have relieved the patient's concern over her heart. In contrast, she became outraged that she was being discharged and reiterated about having to take care of her sick aunt at home. At this point, our sympathy went from the patient to the sick aunt at home. After we personally took her over to the cardiologist in a wheelchair, he heard her story and decided to send her home without a stress test. We disappointed this lady's expectations and sometimes physicians do not make good social workers.

Suicidal patients

These patients are rarely diagnostic dilemmas but frequently pose legal dilemmas for the emergency physician. This is particularly true when the facility does not have psychiatrists on staff and does not have inpatient psychiatry. This is the case with the facility at which we work. Patients whom we feel are at risk of hurting themselves (or hurting others) require an immediate psychiatric evaluation by law. In our case, this entails transferring the patient to a designated psychiatric facility upon medical stabilization. The process of patient transfer is where multiple legal dilemmas arise.

Is the patient willing to accept immediate psychiatric help? Most patients will adamantly refuse this offer of medical help and will need to be involuntarily committed for psychiatric evaluation (i.e. Baker Act). When the emergency physician signs a Baker Act form, hospital security is notified to prevent the patient from leaving the department while the ED staff arranges for patient transfer. Once this is arranged, how is the patient going to be transported? We have always been taught that it should be by law enforcement because they have the authority and ability to prevent the patient from escaping during transit. However, we have encountered many inconsistencies through the years. We have seen the police department refuse to transport at times, deferring the job to the ambulance service. We have also, at times, received resistance from the ambulance service. Finally, what do you do when the family or friends insist on taking the patient? Remember that you are ultimately responsible for the patient's transfer to the psychiatrist.

What about the scenario where the patient is willing to see the psychiatrist immediately and voluntarily? In this event, the ED physician does not fill out a Baker Act form and security is not called to watch the patient. The emergency staff continues to arrange for psychiatric evaluation in the same manner as the patient that is going involuntarily. However, the situation becomes problematic should the patient change his mind before seeing the psychiatrist (including the time spent during transfer). Because the patient has not been involuntarily committed, he can walk away from medical care and carry out his suicidal ideations.

Case 9.13 Things can change any minute

A case in point occurred at our facility recently. A 26-year-old male with no prior medical or psychiatric problems presented to the ED with suicidal ideations. He stated that he had had suicidal ideations every night during the past week including the previous night. He came with his girlfriend and both were extremely concerned that he was going to hurt himself. We told him that we were going to perform a medical evaluation and then arrange for him to receive a psychiatric evaluation at another facility. He thanked us and informed us that he had come to the ED to seek a psychiatric evaluation.

After he was medically cleared and was accepted at the psychiatric facility, we wanted to ask his girlfriend if she felt comfortable with taking him to the center. She left his room and stated that he was now saying that he was fine and that he wanted to go home. Since we were already uneasy about releasing him voluntarily for fear that he would change his mind, these comments convinced us to Baker Act him. However, as we were filling out the form and calling security, the patient told his girlfriend that he was going outside to make a phone call. His cellphone was found on the lawn outside of the ED and he could not be found on the hospital premises. Shortly later, his mother came and was upset that we had let a suicidal patient walk out.

The following hour was a stressful one for everyone in the ED. We called the police to search for a patient who we felt was likely to carry out his suicidal ideations. If successful, the patient's suicide would have been disconcerting not only because it would have meant the end of a youthful, healthy life, but also because it would probably mean a lawsuit for the hospital and the emergency staff that could not be won. Although we did not do anything that was medically incorrect, our fear was that a jury would be emotionally drawn to a grieving mother for her young son's death and how he came to the best place he knew to get help and was not given that assistance. Fortunately for us, the police were able to find the patient at his brother's home one hour later. However, this scenario is not uncommon and will not always lead to a favorable outcome, as in this example.

In a recent article from the *Annals of Emergency Medicine*, it is written that 'most lawsuits about suicide involve patients who have been admitted to inpatient psychiatric units and are brought against the hospital for failing to properly ensure the patient's safety.'[15]

Case 9.14 Is it safe to let go?

The authors of this article also state that they were aware of only one case where an ED physician was found liable for the discharge of a suicidal patient.[15] After planning to admit a depressed and intoxicated 22-year-old male for attempting to kill himself, the physician decided to discharge the

continued

patient after he could not verify that psychiatric care would be covered by the patient's insurance. The patient subsequently committed suicide and the courts found the physician and his employer liable for $240 000. This scenario is not as ridiculous as it may seem. We have seen psychiatric facilities refuse to accept suicidal patients who are uninsured and not committed involuntarily.

Homicidal patients

Treatment of homicidal patients is similar in many ways to that of suicidal patients. The patient's intentions may be occult and may require a high degree of suspicion from the physician in order to be detected. Physicians must make a special effort to protect the safety of these patients or the safety of the people that these patients come into contact with. Remember that although we use the term homicide, protecting the public means prevention of injuries to others and not just the prevention of death to others. Finally, there are legal requirements concerning the reporting of patients who may be suicidal or homicidal.

In contrast to suicidal patients, homicidal patients tend to be more discreet with their intentions. They rarely present with homicidal thoughts as their chief complaint. They are more likely to present seeking treatment for injuries from a fight, an argument, or illicit activity, all of which may instigate the homicidal thoughts. Therefore, physicians should maintain suspicion with particular injuries such as gunshot and stab wounds.

Case 9.15 Duty to protect

Drs Grassie, Henry, and Wagner present a case in *Foresight* where the failure to protect the public led to a settlement.[16] A 24-year-old male came to the ED with a left leg wound and a sketchy history of how it occurred. Both the triage nurse and the ED physician noted that the patient appeared anxious. The wound appeared 'circular, surrounded by a collar of dark, gray-black, sooty material, and seemed to have a front entrance with an exit wound in the back.'[17] The physician commented that it appeared similar to a gunshot wound and told him to stay for some tests. She informed the patient that the tests would be done as soon as possible when he told her that he could not stay long.

The nurse discovered that the patient was not in the room 30 minutes later and informed the physician. She documented this and left the chart to be filed. Another man was brought by ambulance three hours later after getting shot five times. The suspect was the patient seen earlier because he was an acquaintance of the victim and they had just had a drug deal that did not come to fruition. The argument was the main factor in the first shooting.

A lawsuit was filed against the ED physician for failure to report a crime

continued

of violence and negligence in failing to conduct a search when the patient was missing. The authors of this case provide several tips to locating patients that leave the department:
- search the hospital
- page the patient overhead
- notify security
- call the patient or the contacts listed
- call the police.[18]

The ED physician did not document any effort at locating a potentially dangerous patient. This failure did not lead to a good defense and the civil case was settled out of court.

Patients that may require life-saving resuscitation

The emergency department is where a patient who may need life-saving resuscitation is brought. Many of these patients will have suffered a cardiopulmonary arrest at their residence or may be on the verge of cardiopulmonary arrest on presentation to the ED. Therefore, the decision to aggressively treat these patients must be made immediately when the patient arrives in the ED.

Although physicians are trained to treat all patients without a do-not-resuscitate (DNR) order and withhold aggressive measures in those with a signed do-not-resuscitate order, this dogma is frequently more complicated than it seems. Note that what we refer to as 'treat' in these circumstances consists of aggressive life-saving measures such as endotracheal intubation, mechanical ventilation, cardiac defibrillation, etc. Numerous scenarios arise that may be problematic for the treating physician. What if the patient's DNR wishes are not known and the patient is demented or obtunded? If the patient is responsive but is hypoxic, are they considered competent to state their wishes? How about the patient who is accompanied by a family member or friend who does not hold the power of attorney? Can she make a legal decision for the patient? There will also be times when the patient's primary physician will call and ask the ED physician to treat or not treat despite knowing that this decision is not consistent with the patient's DNR status. Should the ED physician comply with the primary physician's orders?

There are also other factors that create difficulty for the emergency physician when making an immediate decision to treat. Patients who come from nursing homes usually arrive with chart records or will have a report called to the hospital prior to their presentation. There are still a number of nursing homes and other less staffed facilities such as assisted living facilities (ALFs) that often may not give a report, send records, or have a DNR status in the patient's chart. In addition, most of these patients are demented or incompetent to verbalize their wishes to the ED physician. They often arrive by ambulance prior to the arrival of any family member or power of attorney. Finally, hospital records are rarely available at the time of the patient's presentation.

Case 9.16 What were the patient's wishes?

This is an example of a difficult case requiring an immediate decision to initiate life-saving treatment. A 96-year-old demented lady from a nursing home was brought to the emergency department for respiratory difficulty and low oxygen saturations at the nursing home. The ED received a report from a certified nursing assistant (CNA) at the nursing home 10 minutes prior to the patient's presentation. The CNA had reported that she could not find any DNR papers in the patient's chart and believed that the patient had full resuscitation wishes. The paramedics gave a similar report to the ED two minutes before the patient arrived.

The patient arrived in severe respiratory difficulty. She was obtunded and had been nasally intubated by the paramedics. Her oxygen saturation was 90% and copious purulent sputum was seen in her oral cavity. The emergency physician made an immediate attempt at oral intubation. This attempt was met with great difficulty due to the patient's copious secretions and multiple attempts were made before successful intubation was achieved. This left the patient with moderate bleeding from her oropharynx from the iatrogenic trauma. The patient's respiratory status stabilized from further decompensation after the intubation.

The patient's son arrived to the ED 10 minutes after her arrival. He witnessed the endotracheal tube and the bleeding in his mother's mouth and was outraged. He exclaimed to the ED staff that his mother had DNR papers at the nursing home and did not want to be on a mechanical ventilator. When the physician and staff explained to him the resuscitation status on her that they were given, he did not believe them. He drove over to the nursing home and obtained the DNR papers and presented them to the emergency staff. He then asked that the tube be removed from his mother's mouth and that she be sent back to the nursing home to 'die.'

Depending on how upset the patient's son was at this incident and how he accepted the explanation of its occurrence, there are many potential legal issues in this case. The above scenario is not uncommon and for the most part unavoidable. The patient and his or her family, however, may view the scenario as unacceptable based on the legal documentation that they have laboriously completed. They may file a complaint against the nursing home for being unprepared and giving false reports. The nursing home may also be accused of hiring personnel who are not appropriately trained and do not comprehend the importance of knowing the patient's resuscitation status or where to find it.

The family may also file a complaint against the paramedics, the emergency physician, and the treating hospital. Despite giving what most of us would agree as appropriate care, an angry patient or family can easily find a plaintiff attorney who can make it appear that this case was handled inappropriately. They may accuse the physician of not making a call to the patient's primary to ascertain the DNR status prior to the patient's arrival. They may also accuse the physician of not reviewing the patient's prior

continued

hospital charts or blame the hospital for not having medical records that can be obtained almost instantaneously (this concept is not far fetched in today's popularization of computerized records). Finally, they may argue that there was time to call the patient's family for this information.

Transportation

Transportation for the emergent patient can sometimes contribute to legal dilemmas. Many patients drive themselves to the emergency department, expect to be treated, and then drive themselves home. Unfortunately, many of the medications that we administer in the emergency department are sedating. Therefore, before we discharge any patient that will be driving, we must ascertain that they were not given anything that was sedating or that there has been adequate time for the medication given to wear off. This protocol must be conscientiously followed because there have been lawsuits against physicians for giving sedative medications to patients who subsequently cause harm to themselves upon ED discharge (whether as an automobile driver or as a pedestrian). Furthermore, there have also been lawsuits from others who were not treated in the ED but received harm from those that were treated in the ED with sedative medications.

The emergency department is a medical setting to which some patients receive a one-way ride with no way of getting home. This scenario occurs, for the majority of the time, in two settings. The first setting is the nursing home patient. Most nursing homes do not have transportation services. The patients that they send are usually on stretchers and are bed-bound. Therefore, it is frequently difficult and time-consuming to find a private transportation service to return these patients to their residence. Consequently, they may stay in the emergency department for hours after discharge and present as a legal risk to the emergency physician in two separate manners. The first manner is the potential to develop medical problems while waiting in the ED (see section above). The second manner is the space and nursing staff that the discharged patients occupy and consume. This leaves fewer resources to treat ongoing patients.

Homeless patients

The second setting where patients frequently come to the ED by ambulance and do not have a means to return is the treatment of homeless patients. These patients are a substantial subset of every ED's census and present as legal risks for many reasons. The ED is the only place to receive medical care for many of them. They often come by ambulance because they have no other means of transportation. In fact, some may come to the ED on a weekly basis during the colder months because they know that they will have a warm and clean bed for a few hours along with a meal. Although they come with a medical complaint (e.g. abdominal pain is the most frequent), they are usually fast asleep before the physician has an opportunity to examine them. This behavior, however, does pose a small legal problem for the emergency physician. Although we may suspect that they are 'crying wolf' for secondary gain, they are also usually medical nightmares waiting to happen. This is because of many factors, including: poor health maintenance, non-compliance with medications, tobacco and alcohol abuse, and poor living conditions. If we do not work them up, there is an increased chance that they may have an acute disease in progress. Even if we do work them up, we still accept the fact that these patients are going to have poorer outcomes in general. However, if the poor outcome comes at the expense of no work-up, a 'caring' plaintiff attorney is always ready to take a case against an 'uncaring physician' or an 'uncaring hospital.'

Homeless patients often come to the ED with a positive 'Samsonite' sign (they bring their luggage with them). This immediately tells the physician that 'I am here to stay.' Hence, they become problematic when the physician attempts to discharge them from the emergency department. They may refuse to leave and even become hostile. Even if the physician has security escort them out, they frequently will hover around the hospital and sign in again to be seen. They may do this repeatedly and make it a test of wills of who is going to concede first. Others will not leave until transportation is provided. We have found that hospitals are usually best off paying for a taxi ride for these patients to a homeless shelter or to their previous destination. Some newspapers may not hesitate to print that 'a patient was kicked out into the street' from a certain facility.

Finally, homeless patients are difficult to treat because of their less than optimal hygiene. On occasions, we have noticed that our local ambulance service brings homeless patients without intravenous access or any other intervention performed en route. When we have a hypotensive patient and we see no attempts at intravenous access, we can only assume that these patients received suboptimal care because of their hygiene. We do not condone these practices and encourage physicians to treat these patients in the same manner as all patients. This means performing the same examinations (including pelvic and rectal exams), ordering the same tests (regardless of cost), and giving the same discharge instructions (although they may not heed the advice) and follow-up appointments.

Liability of consultants

Emergency physicians utilize consultants often and in multiple ways. We sometimes request consultants come to the emergency department to evaluate, treat, and/or admit a patient. At other times, we call a consultant to request the consultant's expertise in their field on a particular patient. Within the latter issue lies one of the most unanswered questions in emergency medicine. Is the advice from a consulting specialist legally binding to the specific patient?

From the ED physician's viewpoint, the answer should be an emphatic: yes! We are trained to recognize and stabilize a large number of disease processes. We are not specialist in any of the traditional fields of medicine (e.g. cardiology, gastroenterology, gynecology, etc.). In fact, emergency departments are designed with call rosters consisting of specialists in all different fields for the emergency physician to obtain help from when he has reached his limitation. This hospital obligation of the consultants is in exchange for maintaining hospital privileges. Therefore, it is from our perspective that the consultants are on medical duty if they are on call and assume medical liability when consulted by the emergency physician. We believe that a clear and unambiguous policy such as this would ensure that ED physicians practice better medicine. If the consultants were not held liable for patients on whom they were consulted but not requested to see, this may discourage ED physicians from seeking medical advice and tempt them to make more critical decisions on their own. Furthermore, if consultants are not held to any legal responsibility, they may instruct the emergency physician to send everyone home without listening to the details of the case.

Starr talks about this subject in his monthly column entitled 'Medicine and the law' in the *Cortlandt Forum* journal.[19] He writes: 'some physicians have been corralled into a legally binding relationship without ever seeing the patient. This occurs whenever the treating physician requests the opinion of a consulting physician. Courts have generally ruled that if the physician being consulted has reviewed the chart, made specific suggestions on the care of the patient, or expected payment for a consultation, then a physician–patient relationship has been established, and the consultant is eligible to be sued for malpractice. On the other hand, cases in which the treating physician has merely talked with the second physician about an aspect of the case are not ruled by this agreement.'[19]

However, ED physicians should be aware that judges and jurors have been very inconsistent on this subject.

Case 9.17 Duty to treat

Selbst and Korin describe a pediatric patient, in *Preventing Malpractice Lawsuits in Pediatric Emergency Medicine*, who presented to the emergency department one week after chest trauma from a football game.[20] He complained of exertional chest pain with occasional shortness of breath, light-headedness, and diaphoresis. The patient had an abnormal EKG about which the ED physician called the cardiology fellow to discuss. The cardiology fellow recommended discharge and did not come to see the patient. Six hours after discharge, the boy was taken to another hospital in cardiac arrest and died. The autopsy revealed myocarditis as the source of the cardiac arrest. An out-of-court settlement was reached against the ED physician and the hospital. The cardiology fellow, however, 'was not included in the settlement; she claimed that she never examined the patient and had no duty to treat him.'[20] Assuming that the ED physician gave an accurate presentation to the cardiology fellow (which is not always the case), the cardiology fellow committed two errors in this case. Patients with blunt cardiac injury and abnormal EKGs should be admitted for monitoring according to Braunwald.[21] The second mistake was claiming that she had no duty to treat the patient. As we stated above, by being on call, she is on official duty through the hospital as a cardiology consultant to the emergency department.

Having stated the above comments, where does the primary care physician fit into the scheme when he or she needs a consultation? The easiest avenue is to consult the patient's own specialist if they already have one. There is already a physician–patient relationship and assuming patient responsibility should not be a problem. If the patient does not already have a specialist but requests a particular one, then this one should be contacted because 'the patient should always come first.' For the cases where the patient does not have specialist and does not request a particular person, the physician can handle it in many different ways. They can choose their favorite specialist, they can choose the specialist that has the most convenient schedule, or they can choose the specialist who is on call at the local hospital. We believe the most diplomatic choice and the one that creates the least liability is the last one. The primary physician should think of his office as a little outlying emergency department without the specialist's service. Whenever these EDs require the consultation of a specialist and/or possible transfer of medical care to this specialist, they usually contact the specialist on call at the nearest urban emergency department. By contacting the physician on call, the referring physician is likely to obtain a specialist who is ready for medical duty (e.g. has not been consuming alcohol with dinner, is not at his daughter's dance recital) and is in a position to offer the best medical care.

Which physician do we call for orders?

There is no single correct answer to this question. Some consultants prefer that primary care physicians or hospitalists admit all patients. Some physicians only have consulting privileges and cannot give admission orders. Admitting physicians for certain diagnoses also vary among facilities (e.g. syncopal patients to be admitted to cardiology versus medicine). Therefore, the choice of admitting physician is affected by multiple factors that are sometimes independent of the patient's medical condition.

The other dilemma with calling physicians for orders comes in the patient who has problems requiring multiple physicians. Is the ED physician responsible for talking to all of the consulting physicians? Again, there is no definite correct answer and each scenario has to be evaluated independently in the best immediate interest of the patient. It is certainly not feasible for the ED physician to present the patient to every physician that is consulted on a patient. On the other hand, admitting physicians are sometimes not familiar with handling acute emergencies that are not related to their field and may need the ED physician to take charge.

Case 9.18 Who are you going to call?

A 79-year-old female came to our ED by ambulance after having a syncopal episode. She had been having abdominal pain with nausea, vomiting, and diarrhea the entire evening before the episode. During the episode, she fell on her left knee and twisted her right ankle. She was not able to bear weight on her legs.

On physical examination, she had diffuse abdominal tenderness without guarding or rebound. Rectal examination revealed tarry stools that were positive for blood. She had moderate swelling and a slight deformity of her left knee. The neurovascular status of the leg was intact.

Emergency department evaluation revealed several significant findings.

continued

She was severely orthostatic and had near syncope when she stood. She had a left bundle branch block on her electrocardiogram. This could not be shown to be old. Her hemoglobin was low at 7 gm/dl. Finally, she had a comminuted and slightly angulated fracture of her left distal femur and a non-displaced spiral fracture of her right lateral malleoli.

After splinting her fractures, we called her primary physician for admitting orders. Her diagnoses were syncope with possible new left bundle branch block, orthostasis, gastrointestinal bleed with anemia, and bilateral lower extremity fractures. We chose to call her primary physician because of two reasons. This physician had a known preference to be called for all of his patients. We also felt that he would be able to coordinate the multi-specialty care that this patient needed and be able to research the chronicity of her abnormal electrocardiogram.

The physician accepted the call and was ready to give admission orders over the telephone. He asked us if we had called the orthopedist and we told him that we would if he wanted us to do so. He replied that he would take care of it. After getting admission orders, the patient was moved to an inpatient bed. We were not aware of her care after she left the ED. The following afternoon, the orthopedist on call called us and asked why he was now getting the consultation. The admitting physician had not seen the patient until the morning and had not consulted the orthopedist until the morning. The orthopedist's frustration was understandable because of the increased swelling and increased difficulty with management of the fracture. It was helpful for us to discover these events because it will change how we manage this primary physician's patients in the future. The orthopedist, however, should also address his concern directly with the admitting physician.

Case 9.19 Can they handle it?

This is another example where the choice of an admitting physician is not easy. A hospital where we worked had a contract with the county sheriff's office to treat all of their inmates. Similarly, the sheriff's office had a contract with a particular physician, in this case a general surgeon, to be the admitting physician for all of their inmates. Consequently, whenever the sheriffs would bring an inmate to the ED that required admission, they would request that the surgeon be called for admitting orders. They were adamant about following this protocol and always stressed this to the ED physician. The surgeon admitted patients with vaginal bleeding, asthma exacerbations, sickle cell disease pain crises, etc. He was a good physician and knew his limitations and used consultants frequently. This was the main reason that we often complied with the requests from the sheriffs. However, this protocol raised certain legal concerns for us.

What would happen if the patient had an adverse outcome while in the hospital and the appropriate specialist was not consulted for the specific problem? Would the ED physician be faulted for not obtaining the

continued

necessary consultant? Remember, the decision of admitting physician was a political one and not necessarily made in the patient's best interest. Are we following the standard of care? Are we practicing cost-effective medicine? Would hospital administration be upset with us if we did not follow the protocol? Would it jeopardize the hospital's contract with the sheriff's office? Unfortunately, there are no simple answers to these questions.

References

1   Guidner G and Leinen A (2003) Subpoenas 101. *EMpulse.* **8**(5): 14–15.
2   Guidner G and Leinen A (2003) Subpoenas 101. *EMpulse.* **8**(5): 14.
3   Guidner G and Leinen A (2003) Subpoenas 101. *EMpulse.* **8**(5): 15.
4   Lowe MR and Mathur P (2003) *A Pocket Guide: legal issues impacting emergency medicine.* Florida College of Emergency Physicians, Orlando, Florida.
5   Edwards FJ (2002) *The M & M Files: morbidity and mortality rounds in emergency medicine.* Hanley & Belfus Inc., Philadelphia, Pennsylvania, 184–5.
6   Selbst SM and Korin JB (2003) *Preventing Malpractice Lawsuits in Pediatric Emergency Medicine.* American College of Emergency Physicians, Dallas, Texas, 111.
7   Edwards FJ (2002) *The M & M Files: morbidity and mortality rounds in emergency medicine.* Hanley & Belfus Inc., Philadelphia, Pennsylvania, 49.
8   Edwards FJ (2002) *The M & M Files: morbidity and mortality rounds in emergency medicine.* Hanley & Belfus Inc., Philadelphia, Pennsylvania, 51.
9   Bamberger JD (2003) HIV postexposure prophylaxis in the emergency department: the morning after is today. *Annals of Emergency Medicine.* **42**(5): 657.
10 Bamberger JD (2003) HIV postexposure prophylaxis in the emergency department: the morning after is today. *Annals of Emergency Medicine.* **42**(5): 658.
11 Edwards FJ (2002) *The M & M Files: morbidity and mortality rounds in emergency medicine.* Hanley & Belfus Inc., Philadelphia, Pennsylvania, 128–9.
12 Edwards FJ (2002) *The M & M Files: morbidity and mortality rounds in emergency medicine.* Hanley & Belfus Inc., Philadelphia, Pennsylvania, 3–5.
13 Edwards FJ (2002) *The M & M Files: morbidity and mortality rounds in emergency medicine.* Hanley & Belfus Inc., Philadelphia, Pennsylvania, 4.
14 Edwards FJ (2002) *The M & M Files: morbidity and mortality rounds in emergency medicine.* Hanley & Belfus Inc., Philadelphia, Pennsylvania, 5.
15 Kennedy SP, Baraff LJ, Suddath RL *et al.* (2004) Emergency department management of suicidal adolescents. *Annals of Emergency Medicine.* **43**(4): 459.
16 Grassie C, Henry GL and Wagner MJ (2004) Interruptions in patient care. *Foresight: Risk Management for Emergency Physicians.* **59**(February): 4–5.
17 Grassie C, Henry GL and Wagner MJ (2004) Interruptions in patient care. *Foresight: Risk Management for Emergency Physicians.* **59**(February): 4.
18 Grassie C, Henry GL and Wagner MJ (2004) Interruptions in patient care. *Foresight: Risk Management for Emergency Physicians.* **59**(February): 5.
19 Starr DS (2003) MI patient suffers the high cost of leaving the ER. *Cortland Forum.* **16**(10): 63.
20 Selbst SM and Korin JB (2003) *Preventing Malpractice Lawsuits in Pediatric Emergency Medicine.* American College of Emergency Physicians, Dallas, Texas, 70.
21 Braunwald E, Zipes DP and Libby P (2001) *Heart Disease: a textbook of cardiovascular medicine* (6e), Vol 2. WB Saunders Company, Philadelphia, Pennsylvania, 1882.

Chapter 10

Other legal issues involving emergency physicians: part 2

- Patient confidentiality
- Aggressive treatment
- Patients who refuse to be evaluated
- Holding patients against their will
- Airway control
- Poisonings or overdoses
- You are in charge of the patient's ED care
- Sometimes you are a primary care physician
- Rape and abuse issues
- Pressures from others about patient flow
- Timeliness of specialty consultations
- Patient complaints
- Worker's compensation issues

Patient confidentiality

Maintaining patient confidentiality is a responsibility of everyone in the medical profession. However, it is a frequent and common problem in the emergency department. The crowded and noisy environment of the ED, along with the sharing of patient rooms and the use of hallway stretchers, creates a setting in which conversations and actions are difficult to keep private. Furthermore, the lack of familiarity between the medical staff and patients facilitates the inadvertent transmission of confidential information.

Patients frequently come to the ED with family and friends who may not necessarily be aware of some aspects of the patient's history. In some cases, the patient may not want others to be aware of her medical problems. Issues that are commonly sensitive to patients include psychiatric, sexual, and social problems. More specifically, histories of suicide attempts, sexually transmitted disease, or substance abuse are frequent reasons for confidentiality lawsuits.

A visit to the emergency department usually draws concerns from the patient's family and friends. There will be a great temptation to provide information to these people when they call to check on the patient's status. This occurs commonly in our facility because we live in a college town and a large percentage of our patients are college students with concerned parents who live hundreds of miles away. However, be cautious that these patients may not always want their medical status known to others. An example common to our practice is the college student who presents to the ED after a motor vehicle accident as a consequence of alcohol intoxication. Her parents will call requesting the status of her condition and the details of the injury. The student, however, does not wish for her parents to be informed of the details of the accident.

Case 10.1 Be careful what you say

Edwards presents a case, in *The M & M Files*, where an emergency physician had good intentions but landed in legal difficulties.[1] A 35-year-old 'frequent flyer' and 'drug seeker' came to the emergency department complaining of a headache. He was well known to the emergency staff but was a new patient to the emergency physician on duty. The ED doctor reviewed the patient's medical and psychiatric records from the past six years. These records detailed a long history of rehabilitation for substance abuse and attempted suicides.

Before examining the patient, the physician encountered the patient's fiancée and attempted to obtain information from her that would help him treat the patient. He inquired whether the patient was still using cocaine (to assess a possible cause of the headache) and mentioned the patient's abuse and mental history in the process. The girlfriend was surprised and upset at these revelations and immediately confronted the patient and terminated her relationship with the patient. The patient filed a complaint against the ED physician with the hospital administration and hired an attorney for legal action. These types of complaint could also be filed for investigation with state health agencies.

We agree with the comments that Edwards make with this case. 'If the same patient was a highly respected judge with the same distant history of substance abuse treatment and suicide attempt, most physicians would be highly sensitive, thoughtful, and circumspect about revealing negative history from a medical record.'[2] 'The best approach lies in the old adage about treating every patient as if he or she were a family member – or a judge, for that matter.'[3]

A special mention has to be made concerning patients with the human immunodeficiency virus (HIV). There are special confidentiality rules that pertain to patients with this virus that are constantly changing. A few years ago, test results for this virus had to be given in person. Now, this rule is being modified where phone results may be allowable but many physicians have not adopted this protocol. It is tough for physicians to keep up with these changes and many state licensing agencies now have continuing medical education requirements concerning HIV reporting.

If you are in doubt, you should err on the side of maintaining patient confidentiality until you have discussed the case with your risk manager or hospital attorney. We had a recent case concerning this issue.

Case 10.2 Some rules are difficult to follow

A 42-year-old transvestite (now a woman) came to our emergency department after a syncopal episode. She had a history of HIV. She was on HIV medications and was under the care of one of the HIV specialists in town. This specialist worked exclusively at a different hospital. The patient had never been to our hospital before.

The triage nurse recorded the patient's medical history in the chart. After reading through it, we walked in to see the patient. She introduced the man in the room with her as her husband. After hearing details of her syncopal episode, we were ready to ask her some questions. One in particular that we wanted to ask was her CD4 count (to assess for opportunistic infection of the brain). As we tried to ask the question, the nurse bumped us and took us out of the room. She informed us that the patient did not wish for her husband to be aware of her HIV status.

This raised immediate concern to us about the health of the patient's husband and the potential for him to acquire a serious virus. The case was discussed with our risk manager who basically told us what we already knew but did not quite agree with. She informed us that we could not discuss the patient's HIV status without her consent. We went back into the room and asked the husband to leave. We strongly encouraged the patient to inform her husband of her health status, especially since they were sexually active. She was aware of the complications of the virus, but adamantly refused. Her reason to not inform her husband was because she believed her husband was cheating on her. This worried us more, due to the potential of the virus to be spread in a mini-epidemic fashion. Our last chance to convince the patient was met with futility. Sometimes the law sure makes it hard to be a physician.

It is important to point out an exception to maintaining patient confidentiality. Emergency physicians frequently treat patients who are brought in by law enforcement or are met in the ED by them. These officers will occasionally ask the physician specific questions about the patient to help them with their report or investigation. As written in Selbst and Korin's *Preventing Malpractice Lawsuits in Pediatric Emergency Medicine*, 'physicians are obligated to cooperate when a crime has been committed.'[4] If a crime has not been committed, however, it may be necessary to keep patient information confidential and inform the police that they may obtain the records by obtaining a formal subpoena.

Aggressive treatment

Emergency physicians perform an extensive number of procedures and engage in numerous other therapeutic modalities. Most are routine and have low complication rates, such as lumbar punctures and reductions or dislocations. Others, such as central venous catheter placement and oral endotracheal intubation carry higher risk and require more skill. Finally, some therapeutic interventions entail significant potential risks and complications. Examples would be thrombolytic therapy for acute cerebrovascular accidents or myocardial infarctions and thoracotomy for the unstable patient with chest trauma.

Although the ED physician's goal is to perform the best therapeutic intervention for her patient, this goal is not always synonymous with the most aggressive therapy. For example, performing a thoracotomy in order to stop a slow ongoing bleed in the chest is likely to create risks that outweigh the benefits. Use of thrombolytics in the emergency department is another intervention that has to be decided with caution. The ED physician must make a thorough assessment of the patient's potential for having a bleeding complication. Furthermore, in the case of acute myocardial infarction, she must also decide whether thrombolytics are even warranted with the increased availability of interventional cardiology in most hospitals today. The decision is best made in consultation with the cardiologist who is inheriting the patient's care. Cardiology consultation is legally paramount in these situations because there are alternative treatment options and because the cardiologist will be treating any potential complication from the intervention.

In the event of an acute ischemic cerebrovascular accident, the use of thrombolytics carries a much lower benefit to risk ratio than its use in acute myocardial infarction. This is because of the numerous factors that are associated with ischemic strokes including:

1 the short time frame from onset of symptoms for initiating thrombolytics
2 the difficulty of patients to pinpoint the onset of their symptoms (since they usually do not have pain as in myocardial infarction)
3 the increased probability of patients having contraindications for thrombolytics (i.e. uncontrolled hypertension, use of other anticoagulants, etc.)
4 there is much less documented benefit of thrombolytic use in acute cerebrovascular accidents than in acute myocardial infarction.

Therefore, it is especially important to consult the neurologist who will assume the patient's care before committing a patient to thrombolytics.

Case 10.3 Treatment that is not without risk

Edwards presents a case, in *The M & M Files,* concerning a gentleman who quickly deteriorated after receiving thrombolytics for an acute ischemic event.[5] A 75-year-old man presented to a small community hospital after the sudden onset of aphasia and right facial weakness one hour prior to presentation. He was a smoker and had a prior history of hypertension. On initial exam, the patient had a blood pressure of 160/97 mm Hg and was confused and had difficulty forming words.

The ED physician ordered a head CT and routine labs, which were all unremarkable. He assessed the patient for any possible contraindications to the use of thrombolytics. He then proceeded to discuss the case with the patient's internist (who evaluated the patient in the ED). The two physicians decided to administer thrombolytics to the patient and the

continued

patient agreed to the consent with the family as witnesses. The patient also had a do-not-resuscitate (DNR) order in his chart.

Upon the completion of the administration of the thrombolytics, the patient was transferred to a general medical floor because of his DNR status. He quickly deteriorated over the next few hours and subsequently died three days later. A second CT scan was never obtained for this patient. This was the initial use of thrombolytics at this hospital and this case brought up several criticisms involving the ED physician and the internist's care. Why was a neurologist not consulted? Why was the patient not transferred to a facility where a stroke team was available? Why was the patient not moved to the intensive care unit? Finally, why was a repeat CT scan of the head not performed?

The treating physicians, in this case, could have also benefited from discussing the treatment options with the patient's family. Since the patient was confused, he was not in an appropriate position to make treatment decisions. Many patients with DNR orders do not wish to have aggressive medical therapy such as thombolytics. Likewise, the families of these patients are also seldom proponents of such therapeutics. These statements are especially true in the case of thombolytics for acute strokes where the risk to benefit ratio is substantial for many patients.

Patients who refuse to be evaluated

We have already discussed the patient who refuses medical treatment and signs out against medical advice. Some patients, however, will only refuse a certain part of the medical evaluation for personal reasons. For example, a lady may feel uncomfortable with a male physician performing a pelvic examination on her or a mother may not want her five-year-old son to get a CT scan to evaluate for appendicitis because of the radiation. Please note that this refusal is distinctly different from a refusal for treatment. These patients still want to be treated; they are just not comfortable with one or more aspects of the evaluation.

As an emergency physician, it is easy to become upset and label these patients as 'difficult' patients and cease the evaluation at this point. However, doing so would not be ethically, medically, or legally wise. Some patients have cultural beliefs or personal experiences that make them hesitant to receive certain medical interventions. For example, we evaluated a child for a persistent cough who had no prior immunizations. His mother did not believe in them because her friend had a child that died after the child had received immunizations. She adamantly refused when we tried to give her child immunizations. Although we were frustrated with her decision, we understood why she felt the way that she did and we proceeded with the evaluation in the usual fashion.

Despite refusing a part of the medical evaluation, a patient that still wants to be treated should still receive as complete a medical evaluation as possible. This could mean offering alternative options (e.g. ultrasound versus CT scan, having a female nurse obtain vaginal swabs, etc.) or choosing more conservative therapy (i.e. admitting the patient, arranging for follow-up evaluation or testing, etc.).

As the physician, you are still medically obligated to do your best to care for these patients.

Similarly, it is in your best legal interest to evaluate the patient as comprehensively as she will allow. Plaintiff attorneys are very skilled at hiring expert witnesses who know all the alternatives that could or should be given to a patient. They will also be able to generate marvelous and credible reasons why their patients refused certain parts of the evaluation and will harp on the fact that their patient still wanted to be treated. Finally, they may take it to the extreme and fault you for 'abandoning' your patient, being inflexible in your medical evaluations, and callous and insensitive to your patient's opinions. In short, they will make you look very bad if you do not show that you did your best to incorporate your patient's wishes into their evaluation.

Case 10.4 Some patients are worth keeping

A 25-year-old morbidly obese female came to our ED at 2 am with right-sided abdominal pain that had been present for two hours. She had nausea but denied fevers, vomiting, diarrhea, urinary or gynecologic symptoms. On examination, she was afebrile and had tenderness in the right side of her abdomen. There was no guarding or rebound and the tenderness was in the middle of the right side. It was not in the right lower quadrant as in the typical area of appendicitis. Likewise, it was not in the right upper quadrant as in the typical area of cholecystitis.

Her abdominal X-ray showed a nonspecific gas pattern without any evidence of gallstones or bowel obstruction. Her urinalysis and urine pregnancy test were both negative. The white blood cell count was elevated at 17 000 cells/microliter. A CT scan of the abdomen and pelvis with contrast was ordered. Shortly later, the CT technician brought the patient from radiology and told us that the patient was refusing her CT.

We went to the patient's room to inquire about this refusal. After explaining our concern for a gallbladder or appendiceal infection, we emphasized that the CT scan was highly recommended. This would not change her mind, as she was adamant about not wanting the procedure. We asked her about 15 times why she did not want the CT, and received the same response every time. 'I just don't want the test!' She would not tell us if she was claustrophobic, afraid of the enema, concerned about the radiation, etc.

Frustrated by her responses, we asked her what she would like us to do for her. She inquired about any alternatives to the CT scan. We told her that we could do an ultrasound but it would be very insensitive for appendicitis because of her size and because of its inherent limitations. She then said that she would just like to go home.

As we went back to the desk to fill out the leaving against medical advice (AMA) sheet, it bothered us that this lady refused a test and did not necessarily refused to be treated. Could we have filled out the alternatives section on the AMA sheet and say that we gave her every alternative? The answer was clearly no. There were alternatives that we could have offered this patient. We could have ordered the ultrasound. We could have asked

continued

the surgeon to evaluate and admit the patient for observation (although this is not likely for a clinically nonsurgical abdomen).

After we realized that there was a substantial likelihood that this patient could have had appendicitis and that alternatives (although poor) did exist, we decided to, one more time, plead our case. We said that we really did not want her to leave and that we felt she really needed the test. Fortunately, she responded, 'Fine, let's get it over with.' The radiologist called us 15 minutes later to tell us that she had early appendicitis. The extra 30 minutes spent in convincing this patient to have a test was fruitful for the patient and for us.

Case 10.5 What are the alternatives?

Edwards presents a case, in *The M & M Files*, where the physician should have offered his patient an alternative when she refused a pelvic examination.[6] A 35-year-old woman came to the ED with intermittent lower abdominal pain for two days. The pain was more prominent on the left side and was not associated with nausea, vomiting, diarrhea, urinary symptoms, or vaginal bleeding. She had had a tubal ligation several years ago and her last period had been a few weeks ago but had been irregular.

On physician examination, the patient had normal vital signs and had 'slight' tenderness in the lower abdomen without guarding or rebound. After obtaining a complete blood count, which was normal, a urine pregnancy test was ordered. When the test was positive, the ED physician recommended to the patient that he needed to perform a pelvic exam. The patient stated that she would prefer to see her family physician (who was female) the following day for the pelvic examination. The ED physician accepted her plan and discharged her.

The patient subsequently had difficulty obtaining a timely appointment with her family physician. The pain grew in great intensity two nights later and was accompanied by a syncopal episode. She was found to be tachycardic and hypotensive on arrival to the ED by ambulance and required fluid resuscitation and immediate surgery after a stat ultrasound showed a probable ruptured ectopic pregnancy. The gynecologist voiced a complaint to the hospital's quality and assurance committee concerning the delayed diagnosis of this patient.

This ED physician did not consider an alternative modality of evaluation when his patient refused a pelvic examination. Namely, in this particularly case, an ultrasound would have been an appropriate test to evaluate abdominal pain in pregnancy. The patient's refusal may seem unreasonable to some emergency physicians (since most emergency physicians are males) but is not at all uncommon. We have encountered this request many times in our practice and have almost grown immune to taking offense to it. In addition, we are always very pessimistic that a patient will be able to see any office physician the following day unless we phone and arrange this with the physician ourselves. This is because medical practices are so

continued

busy these days that it is difficult to accommodate drop-ins. It does not surprise us at all that this patient was not able to see her physician. Finally, for a possible diagnosis such as ectopic pregnancy that has grave consequences if undetected and unaddressed, do not leave the medical fate of these situations to your patient's discretion. The physician must rule out these possibilities to the best of her ability or have the patient sign out against medical advice if the refused examination is required to rule it out.

Documenting that a patient refuses a treatment does not relinquish a physician's liability in the event of a poor outcome. The physician should ensure that all of the proper constituents of the 'against medical advice' (AMA) form have been completed as discussed previously in this book. In addition, the physician should also make every attempt with the patient and her family to convince them to stay, and document these attempts. We have seen many physicians drop their guard whenever they are informed that a patient has refused treatment. As a corollary, an incomplete evaluation increases the opportunity for an adverse outcome.

Case 10.6 It is not over when they leave

Drs Grassie, Henry, and Wagner present a case, in *Foresight*, which emphasizes the importance of good documentation when a patient refuses treatment.[7] A 20-year-old college student presented to the ED complaining of two days of headaches and fevers. She had been to the student health center and was sent over by their physician to 'rule out meningitis.'

On admission to the ED, she did not appear toxic and had normal vital signs with the exception of a 102°F temperature. The ED physician was not impressed with her exam or her clinical appearance and had already performed six negative lumbar punctures that week. A white blood cell count was ordered and was slightly elevated at 12 000 cells/microliter. After her temperature had abated, the physician told the patient and her mother that a lumbar puncture would be needed to rule out meningitis. Both the patient and her mother quickly declined the procedure and the physician did not make any attempt to change their mind. He wrote on the chart, 'lumbar puncture offered, patient refused.'[8]

The patient returned to the student health center the next day because her headache was worse and her temperature was then 104°F. After she had told the physician that she had refused a lumbar puncture, the physician transferred her to another hospital. There, a lumbar puncture confirmed the diagnosis of Streptococcus pneumoniae meningitis. She was left with moderate hearing loss after treatment and her family filed a lawsuit against the initial ED physician.

The initial ED physician did not do several things in his treatment of the patient that would have made this an otherwise easy case to defend. He did not take notice of the patient's headache with a red flag. A headache with

continued

a fever should raise concern for a serious intracranial infection. Furthermore, another physician's impression of the patient's illness was possible meningitis. This physician did not take this impression seriously enough and did not try to convince the patient to have the procedure. He commented that the patient looked like the other patients that he had seen in the week who had had negative spinal taps. This logic is flawed because a patient's health is independent of the health of other patients. Therefore, the probability of this patient having meningitis is not related to the probability of the other patients that the physician had seen earlier during the week.

The plaintiff attorney was quick to emphasize that no AMA form was completed and no alternative treatments were offered. The physician made the jury less sympathetic towards his case when he argued at trial that the AMA form was not a necessity. Whether a physician is right or wrong, it is rarely beneficial to argue against the system to the jury. There was also very little documentation in the chart in terms of the patient's mental status and capacity to make treatment decisions. In addition, there was no record that the risks were discussed with her or of the reason why she refused the test. The physician would have probably had a difficult time defending this case if it was not for the comments of the student health physician. This physician testified that the patient had the mental capacity to make treatment decision during both of her visits with him. The jury subsequently ruled in favor of the defense; however, we believe that the case would have probably never even gone to trial if the proper protocols for refusal of treatment were followed.

Holding patients against their will

We have discussed elsewhere in this book the difficulty in deciding when to hold a suicidal patient against her will. The same or even greater difficulty applies when a patient has a medical condition that may obtund her level of consciousness and ability to make decisions. These situations also require that the treating physician make decisions that are in the best interest of not creating harm to the patient. These decisions, however, are not always consistent with the patient's wishes. They also may vary from case to case and are often best not made by a physician alone. Consultation with another physician, risk manager, or hospital attorney is recommended.

Let us now discuss two similar cases.

Case 10.7 Do not force the issue

Deborah Wear-Finkle, MD, describes a case of false imprisonment in *Medicolegal Issues in Clinical Practice*.[9] A 29-year-old woman, who had a long history of asthma, presented to the ED with an acute exacerbation. Despite stating her wishes of only receiving oxygen, she was given oxygen and

continued

another medication by nebulizer. She became angry when the medication gave her a headache so she took the oxygen mask off and wanted to leave the ED. The treating physician sensed that she was in imminent need of intubation and tried to convince her to stay by offering only conservative therapy. This did not appease her and she decided to go home with her sister. At this point, she was physically restrained from leaving by a security guard and the doctor. The patient was then intubated.

Although the patient's medical condition improved markedly during her hospitalization and she was released from the hospital the following day, she felt traumatized and vowed to never seek help at a hospital again. The patient had another severe asthma attack two years later. She refused to go to the hospital and eventually lost consciousness at home. She was then transported by ambulance to a hospital but died two days later.

The patient's father filed a suit against the initial ED physician and the initial hospital. 'His lawsuit alleged wrongful death, negligence, assault and battery, false imprisonment, and a violation of his late daughter's civil rights. The trial judge instructed the jury that a patient has the right to refuse medical treatment except in a life-threatening emergency situation. The jury found for the defendants.'[9] On appeal, however, the Supreme Judicial Court of Massachusetts reversed the ruling and stated that a patient has the right to refuse treatment even in the event of a life-threatening condition.

Case 10.8 What is sound mind?

We had a very similar case a few years ago. In our case, a 55-year-old woman with severe chronic obstructive pulmonary disease (COPD) presented to our ED with an acute exacerbation. She was extremely hypoxic on arterial blood gas with an arterial oxygen pressure of 52 mm Hg on two liters of oxygen. She was also struggling to breathe with pursed breathing and a leaning forward position. Although she appeared slightly lethargic, she was able to converse with us with full comprehension when awakened. She made it perfectly clear that she did not want to be hospitalized for her breathing. However, we did not feel comfortable honoring this request because, as in the situation in the previous case, she was on the verge of intubation. We consulted the internist on call to see her. After seeing the patient, the internist had similar concerns as we did. Upon consulting with risk management, the physicians involved decided that involuntary hospitalization was in the best interest of the patient and that the patient's hypoxia was a justification to consider her ability to make decisions to be impaired. We also took into consideration that the patient lived almost an hour away from the nearest hospital and that she would probably not survive a release from the ED.

In our case, however, the patient was able to avoid intubation and did well during her hospitalization. She still stated that she was upset with the hospitalization but no complaint was filed and the outcome was probably the best for everyone involved. However, the outcome of this case could have been similar to that of the previous case.

Case 10.9 Work till you die

Finally, we had a remarkable case at the Veterans Administration Hospital of a patient who left against medical advice. A 52-year-old male with a history of heavy tobacco use and hypertension came to the ED with two days of shortness of breath, productive cough with yellow sputum, and tightness across his chest. He had no history of asthma or coronary artery disease but had audible wheezing without a stethoscope and was bent over with pursed breathing. He could barely talk yet joked when asked if he was a smoker. He responded that 'I will quit in 10 minutes.' His oxygen saturation was 97% on room air and his arterial oxygen pressure on blood gas was 68. We ordered some labs that showed an EKG with new q waves in the precordial leads that were not previously present, and a CPK value of greater than 2000 U/L. The chest X-ray and troponin, however, were normal.

After a couple of nebulizer treatments, intravenous steroids, and nitroglycerin, the patient's breathing was minimally improved and the chest tightness remained. We told the patient that he needed to be admitted because his breathing was not better and that he could be having a heart attack. He stated that he could not stay because he would lose his job if he missed work tomorrow. After we stressed repeatedly that he could die before then or would be a danger to himself and others while performing his duties as a cab driver, he responded, 'I would rather die than be homeless.'

After he signed the form to leave against medical advice, he heard that the patient in the adjacent bed was being discharged. Because he could barely muster a voice, he asked his nurse to ask that patient if he needed a ride home because our patient was a cab driver and he needed the business. The nursing staff laughed at this gesture and the patient told them that his mother taught him to always maintain humor even in periods of distress. He added that his mother told a joke right before she died. We strongly advised him not to drive but we had no legal means to keep him. We treated him to the best of our ability with steroids and inhalers and hoped that he would not cause any harm to himself or to others. He left the ED in discomfort but was smiling and shaking everyone's hand.

Airway control

Providing an airway for a patient and protecting it are two of the most important duties of the emergency physician. Some patients will have an obvious need for an airway. These include patients in cardiopulmonary arrest, patients with respiratory failure, patients with refractory seizures, and patients with anaphylaxis. Other patients will not have an immediate need for an artificial airway but will need one for other anticipated reasons. These include patients who will be transferred (to CT or another facility), patients at high risk for aspiration (head injuries, cerebrovascular accidents), and those with the potential of losing their airway (inhalation injuries, epiglottitis). For most of these latter cases, the emergency physician should provide an artificial airway if there is any concern that the airway will be lost.

Case 10.10 Do not risk losing

Edwards presents a case, in *The M & M Files*, where the failure to perform a prophylactic intubation led to a complaint against a physician.[10] A 56-year-old woman with a history of hypertension was brought to the ED after developing a sudden headache, nausea, and left-sided weakness. On arrival, she was flaccid on her left side and was responsive only to painful stimuli. The patient was taking her own breaths and they were not agonal so the ED physician transported her directly to the radiology suite to get a head CT.

As the patient was on the CT table (where a large intracerebral hemorrhage was seen), she seized, vomited, and went into arrest. She was intubated with difficulty and transferred to surgery. She eventually recovered despite suffering aspiration pneumonia and acute respiratory distress syndrome. The radiology director filed a complaint against the ED physician for transporting a comatose patient without first protecting the airway. The ED physician replied that the patient did not need intubation in the emergency department but then realized that he should have protected the patient's airway given the decreased airway reflexes from the central nervous system injury.

Case 10.11 Too tight and secure

On the other end of the spectrum, we read a case a few years ago about a physician who received a lawsuit because he intubated a patient. An eight-year-old boy was brought to the ED after suffering significant second degree burns to his trunk and inhalation injuries during a house fire. The ED physician felt that this child met the criteria and would be better treated at a burn center. After discussing the case with the center, the arrangements were made for helicopter transport. The physician was concerned about the inhalation injury causing progressive edema to the boy's airway. He decided to intubate the child with an appropriate size ET tube with a cuff.

The boy was intubated without problem and the cuff was inflated. Transport to the burn center went smoothly and the boy received excellent burn care. His hospital course, however, was complicated by the development of subglottic stenosis from the cuffed ET tube and the boy received permanent injury to his larynx. The parents filed a lawsuit against the initial ED physician. The physician was faulted despite protective and good intentions for the child's health. At the age of eight, it is somewhat difficult to decide whether to use a cuffed ET tube or not based on the size of the larynx. What if the child was not intubated and lost his airway during the flight? Would the outcome have been much worse for the child's health? As we can see from these two cases, the decision on when to intubate is not always as easy as it seems.

Poisonings or overdoses

Poisonings and overdoses frequently have legal implications. They may occur as a result of suicidal or homicidal plans. They may also be associated with child or elderly abuse. Finally, they may result in a disabling or fatal insult in an otherwise healthy person. Therefore, care for these patients must be done with meticulous detail and documentation to avoid future legal scrutiny.

Fortunately, poisonings is one area of emergency medicine where there is easily available assistance. There are poison control centers in every state that are available for consultation 24 hours a day. They can provide a wealth of information concerning symptoms, treatment, and observation of these patients. The facilities are equipped with treatment protocols for many specific poisonings. They also have an on-call toxicologist who can give consultation. Their staff are also excellent in calling back to check on patients.

Many physicians are not aware of the services of the poison control center. Although many emergency physicians utilize the center, some ED physicians and many primary care physicians do not. In addition, poison control centers are also helpful for other situations such as snakebite envenomation and toxic inhalants or exposure (e.g. chemical exposure to the eye). We strongly believe that most, if not all, poisonings or overdoses in the emergency department should be treated with a consultation to the poison control center. They will be your best legal defense in court in the case of a poor outcome.

Case 10.12 Poisoning the mind

Edwards presents a case, in *The M & M Files*, where a poisoning of a patient became a legal matter.[11] A young man came to the ED with paint covering his beard and stating that he was feeling ill after 'huffing' paint fumes. Although he had normal vital signs, the triage nurse documented that he had slurred speech and was 'not highly oriented.' Consequently, she took him to a monitored bed, pulled the rails up, and informed the ED physician.

The ED physician listened to the nurse's comments and proceeded with the stack of charts of patients that were waiting to be seen. The patient felt better 20 minutes later and wanted to leave through the ambulance entrance. A different nurse stopped him and escorted him back to his room. She then immediately informed the ED physician. The physician was occupied with a laceration and told the nurse to have him sign out against medical advice. The patient signed an irregular line and left the ED. His chart was flagged on review the next day because of the uncertainty of the patient's competency to decline medical treatment. He could not be reached at the telephone number that he had left. He became lost to follow-up.

This scenario is not uncommon in the emergency department. The ED physician is managing multiple patients at a time. It is tempting and convenient in a busy department to have a patient sign out and relieve the physician of any medical and legal liability. However, 'out of sight does not always mean out of mind.'

This is especially true in cases of poisoning. Did the intoxication prevent the patient from making sound medical decisions for himself? What if he had been intoxicated with other gases or drugs? Could a medical condition such as stroke be causing the patient's mental status change? Was the inhalation a deliberate attempt at killing himself? It is easy to see from these questions that the ED physician and the hospital's responsibility to the patient did not end when the patient signed the AMA form. The ED physician failed by not evaluating the patient immediately at the point of care and determining whether he was mentally competent to sign the form or whether he should be kept against his will for a medical evaluation.

You are in charge of the patient's ED care

The emergency department is a multi-specialty arena. Physicians from virtually all specialties treat patients in the ED. The ED physician is involved in the care of every patient there (with the exception of the patient who is a direct admit and waiting for a bed). Most of the time, the interactions and decisions of the physicians involved in the patient's care will be in accord with each other. There will be times, however, when a consulting physician will alter or cancel a recommendation by the ED physician. As the ED physician, you must determine for yourself whether you are comfortable with these decisions.

When the patient is in the emergency department, you bear the largest responsibility for them. If you feel strongly that something needs to be done, then you should do it regardless of another provider's opinion. Remember that, although consultants are experts in their fields, no one is used to seeing as many emergencies as you are. Therefore, stick with your decisions and your gut instincts. Also, do not leave tasks that you can perform in the ED undone and assume that another physician will do them. Why take chances when it is much better to take control? We will give two examples that we frequently see in our practice.

The first involves a patient who is found to be anemic. If the anemia is worse or new, then the physician should perform a rectal exam and get a rough idea if the patient is having a gastrointestinal bleed. We have seen many physicians refer patients for outpatient testing or admit patients for further testing without performing this simple and quick test. Why wait days or weeks to get a hemoccult card result or a gastrointestinal evaluation when a plaintiff attorney will be sure to ask you if you have fingers?

The second example is the patient with shortness of breath. We will often admit these patients for diagnoses that we discover in the ED evaluation such as congestive heart failure, pneumonia, asthma exacerbation, etc. Many of these patients will also have multiple risk factors for pulmonary embolus, which will be left for the admitting physician to address. We have seen patients discharged after a hospital admission for shortness of breath where an evaluation of pulmonary embolus was not ordered and the patient was subsequently found to have one.

Case 10.13 Stand firm

Tanya Albert presents a case, in *American Medical News*, about a lawsuit that could have been prevented had the ED physician stood his ground.[12] A $5 million dollar jury award was recently found against three physicians for failing to detect child abuse in a prompt fashion. A babysitter brought an infant to his pediatrician after the baby had fallen and hit his head. The pediatrician did not notice any signs of trauma and the boy appeared alert and neurologically normal. Since there was nothing else to suggest child abuse, the pediatrician sent the child home and instructed the mother to call if any problems arose.

Later that night, the boy's father came home and agreed with his wife that their child was not acting like usual. After talking to their pediatrician, the physician instructed them to go to the ED. The parents had the understanding that they were going to the ED to get a head CT scan for their child. The ED physician examined the infant and described him as 'playful, bright and engaging.' He ordered a CT scan of the head and called the on-call pediatrician to see the child. The on-call physician noted that the child was 'alert and active.' Even the ED nurse said that the boy was 'playful and active.'

The pediatrician cancelled the CT and discharged the child home and instructed the parents to follow up with his pediatrician in a couple of days. When they did, the pediatrician also did not notice anything wrong with the child. About three weeks later, the babysitter called the child's mother at work and told her that the infant was unresponsive and lying on the floor. The child was flown by helicopter to a medical center for emergent surgery of a massive subdural hematoma that was caused on the same day. The babysitter was charged and found guilty of child abuse.

The neurosurgeon also mentioned the presence of a small subdural hematoma that was days to weeks in duration; the parents filed a lawsuit against the three physicians for failure to diagnose child abuse and the injuries that were a result of it. The physicians were found negligent by not ordering a CT scan sooner and the large award was given in favor of the parents of the disabled child.

Although it may never be known for certain if the child had significant (or any) injuries during the initial visits with the three physicians, the physicians lost the suit because they did not take notice of some red flags in the case. This failure of recognition made the exact time that the serious injuries occurred irrelevant. Remember in Chapter 4 when we described tips from Dr Ramon Johnson on preventing errors in pediatric practice. The second 'red flag' that he presented was to take parents seriously when they say that there has been a behavior change in their child. The physicians should have also recognized that repeat physician visits are usually futile unless there is a step-up in care. Finally, the on-call pediatrician had to explain in court why he canceled the head CT and the ED physician had to tell why he did not push for it if he had ordered it.

Sometimes you are a primary care physician

Emergency physicians see a significant number of urgent care and non-urgent care visits annually. There are multiple aspects of our healthcare industry that contribute to this problem. Patients on managed healthcare plans cannot see their physician because the provider's schedule is full. Other patients do not have physicians or are uninsured and the ED is their only means of getting medical treatment. Some patients are too embarrassed to go anywhere else (e.g. sexually transmitted disease check). There may be a shortage of specialists in the area (e.g. dentist, dermatologist) necessitating a prolonged wait for an appointment. Finally, some patients just cannot wait to see their own physician.

For whatever reason, non-emergent visits to the ED have become the standard and not the exception. In fact, most moderate to large size EDs have now installed 'express care' or 'fast track' centers in order to see these patients and maintain the availability of beds in the main ED for emergent patients. The income generated by these centers has become profitable for most emergency physician groups. In fact, many EDs advertise their urgent care services in order to attract more business. Therefore, we will probably be seeing an increasing number of 'primary care visits' in the ED in the future. One particular patient visit that we will always remember as a classic 'primary care' type visit occurred a few years ago. A middle-aged man was supposed to go the laboratory to have a fasting cholesterol drawn at 7 am when the place opened. At 6 am, he decided that he could not wait any longer and signed into the ED to have it drawn. That was one extremely high priced blood draw!

With the increasing number of 'primary care' visits, emergency physicians will be expected to act more like primary care providers and assume more responsibility for the follow-up of these patients. How many times in our careers have we told a patient that 'we cannot do much more for them and that they need to see their own physician?' Patients, and the public, do not realize sometimes that our training is limited to emergent medical conditions and, similarly, our tests are designed to detect emergent conditions. We have limited training at cancer screening, managing chronic medical conditions such as hypertension and diabetes, and treating chronic pain. Patients who do not have anywhere else to go, however, still rely on the ED to manage these problems. Lawsuits and complaints have arisen whenever suboptimal treatments have resulted.

Case 10.14 Nowhere else to go

Edwards presents a case, in *The M & M Files*, where a complaint was made against an ED physician for not giving adequate disposition instructions.[13] The case pertains to a patient with a dental complaint. Dental complaints are common in the ED and most ED physicians do not have extensive training in dental care. Furthermore, most EDs do not have adequate dental emergency coverage or equipment (e.g. panorex X-ray for dental trauma). Fortunately, there are very few dental emergencies. Therefore, we treat most patients with dental pain supportively with antibiotics and pain medicines and instruct them to follow up with a dentist. Patients often cannot do this,

continued

however, because of the scarcity of dental appointments available and the lack of financial resources. Therefore, the ED physician is likely to become their 'primary physician' when they return to her with the same complaints. You cannot just turn them away in this circumstance and you are expected to figure out a solution. We will give examples after presenting Edward's case.

A 49-year-old homeless man came to the ED complaining of tooth pain and facial swelling for two weeks. He had no fevers or compromise of his airway. He had swelling of the angle of his mandible on the right but no tenderness of his teeth on that side. His general dentition was poor with numerous missing teeth and decay of the remaining teeth. The ED physician made the diagnosis of a dental abscess and discharged the patient on penicillin and acetaminophen with codeine. He also recommended that the patient follow up with a dentist but offered no other specific discharge instructions.

Over a month later, an otolaryngologist called the ED director to complain because he had diagnosed the patient with pharyngeal carcinoma. The patient had been referred to him just a few days earlier by a dental clinic. He was upset with the delay time that it took to make the diagnosis and that this delay was going to make the prognosis worse.

In the practice of emergency medicine today, you frequently need to assume that anyone who does not have a primary doctor is unlikely to follow up with anybody. Therefore, pretend you are their primary physician and make sure that you give strict discharge instructions. For this patient who has already developed an abscess, it may have been helpful to instruct him to find a dentist as soon as possible. If you do have a dentist on ED call, you may try to contact that person to arrange an appointment. If you do not, or the patient does not have the financial resources to see one, find out if the free clinics in town have dental services (many of them do). In addition, because this patient is unlikely to follow up with anyone in the near future, you should make it clear when they should return to see you. In this way, you may be able to prevent a worsening problem from turning into a disaster. Finally, the status of this patient's dentition probably warranted the ED physician to comment on it and address it. We mentioned above that ED physicians are not the best at detecting cancers and we understand why the diagnosis of pharyngeal carcinoma was not made in this case on the first visit. However, the abnormality and inconsistency of the patient's physical exam justified a recommendation for him to see a dentist as soon as possible.

Case 10.15 Another time and place

Another example from *The M & M Files* of expectations of primary care in the emergency department involves a healthy 29-year-old woman.[14] The young lady presented to the ED with several days of fever, nausea, headache, muscle, and joint aches. She was not taking any medications and

continued

denied any sore throat, cough, vomiting, or diarrhea. Her physical exam was normal with the exception of a temperature of 100.1°F. The ED physician discharged the patient with a 'viral illness' and did not give her any specific follow-up instructions.

Over the next six days, the patient's symptoms became progressively worse. She went to a primary care office where multiple tests were ordered. The results of the test suggested that the patient had rheumatoid arthritis. The primary physician encouraged her to file a complaint against the emergency department and contest its bill.

From the events of this case, it is apparent that not only does the public expect us to provide primary care in the ED but some physicians also expect the same. In our years of practice, we would say that most emergency physicians would have treated this patient the exact same way in the ED. A young and healthy individual without a focus of acute serious infection should probably be treated symptomatically initially. Further tests may be needed if there is no improvement or the symptoms become prolonged. The ED would lose much of its proficiency and income if we were to order tests on every patient with the above symptoms.

Unfortunately, you often only get one chance to make a good impression in the ED. While your focus is on detecting and treating acute and emergent conditions, the public and, sometimes, their primary physician see the ED as a medical arena where there is an infinite range of diagnostic tests and consultants available. In the above example, most ED physicians would not consider rheumatoid arthritis a diagnosis that should be made in the ED. It is regarded as a 'zebra' diagnosis in emergency medicine, usually requires confirmation tests that are not available during the initial visit, and does not require emergent therapy. Therefore, the primary physician was inappropriate to find fault with the ED physician for missing the diagnosis. Furthermore, she likely ordered confirmation tests that took several days for the results to return.

The final note is that we rarely diagnose anyone as having a 'viral syndrome.' This has become too much of a catch-all phrase and lawyers will 'eat you up alive' if you are wrong. It is better to use the term 'possible viral syndrome' or anything that is less exclusive because there are many entities (e.g. bacterial infections, autoimmune diseases, drug reactions, etc.) that may mimic viral syndromes.

Rape and abuse issues

Rape and abuse are two components of forensic medicine that are not uncommon in emergency medicine. The politically correct term for rape is 'sexual assault' and is recommended in legal documentation. Abuse is a broad term and incorporates child abuse, elderly abuse, domestic abuse, and sexual abuse. Rape can be considered as a subset of abuse. Therefore, we will use the general term abuse in the remainder of this section.

Some patients of abuse will present overtly and seek help. Other patients will have vague complaints and require detective work and a suspicious mind on the part of the clinician. Any potential clues that are missed by the clinician are considered inexcusable so the physician must err on the side of protective treatment. Although some will welcome medical and legal help, others may shun assistance. Confidentiality and safety issues are frequently vital to the care of these patients. Finally, laws concerning the reporting of these cases exist and may vary between states. Therefore, it is apparent that patients of abuse are frequently challenging to treat.

In our practice, we treat abuse patients in a slightly similar manner as we treat the patient with a poisoning. Some of the same legal implications that were discussed under 'Poisonings or overdoses' above also apply to the abuse patient. We try to follow the treatment guidelines of the 'experts' just as we do with poisonings.

For patients of a sexual assault, the history and physical exam must be performed with thoroughness and consistency. These cases have an inclination to be brought to court and reviewed by others. Documentation must be accurate enough to jar your memory years from now if you are subpoenaed. Some EDs will have a designated sexual assault nurse examiner (SANE) who is experienced and skilled at these exams. For those that do not, we recommend that the case be discussed with the sexual assault unit of the local sheriff's office. They will usually come out to the patient and provide tips on collecting data. Remember that the treatment of a sexual assault is multifactorial. It does not only include evaluating and treating any physical problems of the assault, but also prevention of sexually transmitted diseases, counseling of emotional stress, protecting the patient from further harm, and ensuring proper follow-up and further testing.

Patients of other forms of abuse are handled in a similar fashion. Report cases to the proper authorities and follow their protocols. Elderly abuse is reported to the elderly abuse hotline and child abuse is reported to the Department of Children and Families in our practice.

Case 10.16 Suspicious mind required

Edwards presents a case, in *The M & M Files*, where the signs of child abuse did not raise the suspicion of an ED physician.[15] An eight-year-old infant was brought to the ED by a couple at midnight after the child had 'stopped breathing.' The couple was young and this was their first child. The event occurred around 10 pm while the mother was at work and the father was alone with the child. It lasted approximately one minute and was not associated with any seizure activity.

Although the physical exam and the vital signs were essentially unremarkable, the physician noted that the child was 'somewhat lethargic, might be sleeping.'[16] He also found bruises on both sides of the child's chin. A chest X-ray was unrevealing and the child was observed for an hour. During this time, the child became more active and alert. He was discharged and the parents were instructed to see his pediatrician for any further problems.

The mother noticed a worsening of the child's condition by the morning and noted that he would not eat. She took him to the emergency department of a children's hospital. A head CT showed an intracranial bleed. He was also discovered to have several bruises on his back and retinal and vitreous hemorrhages. The child was admitted, stayed in the hospital for two weeks, then was discharged into foster care. His father, meanwhile, confessed to abusing the child and was arrested. The first ED physician was reprimanded by the state health agency for poor documentation, failure to initiate further testing, and not protecting the child.

The finding of bruises on a child should always raise a physician's suspicion for child abuse. At a minimum, the physician should ask for the cause of the bruising. Additionally, it is prudent to completely undress the child or perform a more extensive evaluation for further signs of abuse.

In this particular case, there were other red flags that were disregarded. The child was alone with one parent when the episode occurred. The parents were young and this was their first child. The patient's symptoms were atypical and were associated with lethargy. These should have prompted a more thorough evaluation than a chest X-ray and an hour's observation.

When a child has a delayed presentation for an injury, child abuse should be suspected until proven otherwise. We usually discuss these cases with the Department of Children and Families and let them make the decision of further investigation. Although abusive parents may provide reasonable explanations, it is never customary to delay the care of one's child when she needs it.

Case 10.17 Not nice to wait

The following example from Selbst and Korin's *Preventing Malpractice Lawsuits in Pediatric Emergency Medicine* highlights this rule.[17] Several days after dropping his two-year-old daughter from a height of six feet, a father brought his child to the ED for vomiting and joint stiffening. The man said that he did not seek treatment earlier because he was afraid of telling his wife of the event. The ED evaluation revealed that the child had a small intracranial bleed but she was not admitted. A week later, the child was admitted for worsening symptoms and found to have skull fractures and significant brain injury as a result of shaken baby syndrome. A settlement of $3.7 million was awarded against the medical center for the failure to detect and report child abuse.

Some physicians are concerned about their legal liability with making an incorrect diagnosis of abuse. According to the numerous books that we have read and the many people with whom we have spoken, the physician is generally immune from legal repercussions if she has a genuine concern for the safety of the patient and takes measures to protect this safety. The patient's party may file a lawsuit or a complaint with the state health agency (as in our case with the suicidal patient). However, the physician will eventually be exonerated.

Case 10.18 Report any doubts

Selbst and Korin present such a case in *Preventing Malpractice Lawsuits in Pediatric Emergency Medicine*.[18] After examining a five-year-old girl who was brought in for bloody stools and constipation, an ED physician suspected sexual abuse and reported the child's parents to the Bureau of Child Welfare. The judge agreed with the physician's assessment and ordered that the child be taken from her parent's custody. The parents filed a malpractice lawsuit for misdiagnosis against the physician that was to no avail as the courts cited that the physician 'acted in good faith and was immune from liability.'

Pressures from others about patient flow

We mentioned in other areas of this book about the overcrowding problems of the emergency department. Because of this, ED physicians receive pressure from nurses, ED managers, their physician group, and hospital administration to keep patients moving in and out. Almost every ED keeps track of various times. These include the time for a patient to be triaged, the time for a patient to be brought to the ED, the time the patient waits to see a physician, and the total time that is spent in the ED.

While it is important to be an efficient and productive physician in the ED, the medical care rendered is the most important concern and must not be compromised. Remember that while the pressure groups above may pat you on the back or reward you with bonuses for being the most productive physician, they also will likely be the first to look away when you are hit with a malpractice suit. In addition, our goal should always be to do what is best for the patient and not for us or for others.

Case 10.19 No right to complain

Edwards presents a case, in *The M & M Files*, where an ED physician received criticism for ordering tests that he felt his patient needed.[19] A 64-year-old woman came to the ED with teeth pain. She had had the pain for one week but denied any medical problems. Her left molar was tender and the physician was about to discharge her with a prescription for penicillin when he noticed that the nurse had written irregular pulse on the triage sheet.

The physician decided to ask the patient more questions and discovered that she had recent weight loss, malaise, and polydipsia and polyuria. An EKG showed a multifocal atrial tachycardia rhythm while blood work revealed a hemoglobin level of 8.8 mg/dl and a blood glucose level of 290 mg/dl. He then contacted the patient's physician and arranged for her to have an appointment and further testing the following day. The nurse manager of the emergency department complained to the medical director

---

continued

the following day why a patient who came in for teeth pain was kept in the ED for over three hours and received extra tests.

Emergency physicians deal with complaints like these frequently. While a few have merit and do serve to improve the physician's future performance, most are unjustified after a physician reviews them further. In our opinion, only a physician can understand what another physician's thought process is during a medical encounter. This thought process cannot be adequately evaluated by other staff members such as nurses, managers, or administrators. Would you expect a paralegal to understand what an attorney is thinking?

The physician's actions in this case were not only understandable but also commendable. He was keen enough to review the patient's vitals and read the nurse's notes. He recognized the potential association of acute coronary syndrome with dental pain. In the presence of an abnormal rhythm without a prior history of such, an electrocardiogram is mandatory. Failure to detect the new presence of atrial fibrillation or heart block can lead to strokes and sudden cardiac death.

When the physician obtained the further history of weight loss, malaise, polydipsia, and polyuria, these symptoms warranted bloodwork for several reasons. Was the patient anemic? Did she have an electrolyte imbalance? Could she possibly be in diabetic ketoacidosis? All three of these could potentially represent emergencies that need to be immediately detected. By taking the time to ask a few more questions, ordering a couple of basic laboratory tests, and talking with the physician's primary physician, the ED physician placed the patient in a position to have several medical conditions investigated and treated. Specifically, this patient may have had chronic obstructive pulmonary disease (suggested by multifocal atrial tachycardia), diabetes (suggested by blood sugar and symptoms), and cancer (suggested by anemia and weight loss). Are we fair in saying that this was worth spending three hours in the emergency department?

Timeliness of specialty consultations

When is the perfect time to consult a specialist? This has been a dilemma for emergency physicians that will probably never be answered with a consensus. There are certainly many factors that are involved in the decision to call a consultant. It depends on the ED physician's comfort level and experience with handling the particular problem. It also depends on the ED physician's experience with previous interactions with the consultant. For example, a consultant who has a long history of reluctance to come in may want more definitive evidence of a medical condition before coming. In contrast, ED physicians may not hesitate to call a consultant who is always friendly and ready to help. It may be easy to say that personal attitudes should not interfere with professional work but, in reality, they always will and cannot be eliminated from any profession. In some situations, a physician may wait for a particular test before calling the consultant (in correspondence with the standard of care), but there may be unexpected delays in obtaining the tests. (Please see Chapter 8 under 'Equipment failure' and 'Prolonged waiting times'.)

For the plaintiff attorney, there is only one correct answer to the leading question of this section. The correct time to call a consultant is the time when the patient's injury could have been prevented. If the emergency physician called the consultant 10 minutes after the patient arrived, that was one minute too late. Equipment failure and other intangibles that are difficult for us to control are not acceptable. Plaintiff attorneys are skilled experts at emphasizing crucial time lapses to a jury. Hence, in order to counter these tactics, a defense must have thorough documentation of the justification for these time lapses.

Case 10.20 A matter of timing

As an example, we will use a particular case from Selbst and Korin's *Preventing Malpractice Lawsuits in Pediatric Emergency Medicine*.[20] A 17-year-old girl was brought to the ED after an automobile collision with a building. The girl's vital signs remained stable and the ED physician called the surgeon 1½ hours after her arrival to evaluate the patient. Two hours later, she died during surgery from massive internal hemorrhage caused from lacerations to her aorta, spleen, and hepatic vein.

A lawsuit was filed against the ED physician and the hospital for the delay in calling in the surgeon. The defense's argument was that the timing of the call was appropriate, given the stability of the patient's vital signs. They also felt that the severity of the girl's injuries made it irrelevant as to when she was taken to surgery. The jury's vote was split but the case was settled after the trial with the ED physician paying the entire settlement.

Documentation is the key to defending cases like this one. Stable vital signs are only one of many criteria to determine the extent of traumatic injuries. Did the patient have any significant abdominal tenderness? If so, the surgeon should be called immediately or a rapid diagnostic test for abdominal trauma such as a focused abdominal sonographic exam should be performed. Sometimes, the mechanism of injury and the extent of damage to the car alone warrant a call to the surgeon. Was there external evidence of internal hemorrhaging such as Cullen's sign or Grey Turner's sign? Did the physician perform pelvic and rectal exams to search for bleeding or document the presence and strength of pulses in the lower extremities. A physician who does a thorough job of documenting all of these other factors would probably be justified in delaying the call to a surgeon for 1½ hours. Emergency physicians treat many patients from automobile accidents and the shortage of general surgeons makes it impossible to call them to evaluate every trauma immediately. On the other hand, if a thorough history and physical is not performed or the documentation is poor, then the timing of the consultation will always be too late.

Patient complaints

Patients are consumers and they have the right to voice or write complaints if they are not satisfied with their care. Patient complaints, when valid, help us improve our practice. We must take the time to listen to or read each complaint as objectively as we can. We cannot adopt the 'I can't be wrong' attitude because we will never get better and will surely fail. Some complaints, however, are not based on physician error. They are sometimes made out of patient frustration or for secondary gain. Some patients are aware of the legal crisis in medicine and are not hesitant to exploit it to their advantage.

Case 10.21 Missed but considered and treated

We saw a 21-year-old male after a rollerblading accident in which he ran into a car. He came to the ED by ambulance and was in full spinal immobilization. He complained of numerous areas of pain and received numerous X-rays. We read all of the X-rays as negative. Although we did not see a fracture of his left wrist, one was suspected because he had tenderness in his anatomic 'snuff box.' Therefore, we gave him pain medicine in the ED and placed him in a thumb spica splint. He was given a prescription for pain medicine and instructed to follow up with the orthopedist in one week for an occult fracture. He was also told to follow up sooner if his pain worsened.

When we came back on shift four days later, we received the radiology report of the patient's left wrist. There was a non-displaced intra-articular fracture of his distal radius. We, along with the ED director, could not see the fracture on initial review. Then we magnified the digital image by 3–4 times and were able to see it. We called the patient to inform him of this but figured that it would not have changed his management.

The patient was furious with us when we told him of the fracture. He said that his pain had become worse and he had seen the orthopedist two days ago. The orthopedist had informed him of the fracture. He repeatedly made false claims that we told him that there were no fractures. Over the next few days, he made daily calls to the hospital administration, the ED director, and ED manager to complain about his care. Using hostile tone and language, he accused us of missing the fracture, placing the splint too tight, not giving him pain medicines in the ED, and making him wait too long for treatment. He threatened to file a malpractice suit unless his ED bill was dropped.

Although we are biased in this case because of its personal nature, we felt that the patient was trying to exploit us for secondary gain. The fracture was missed on radiograph but not clinically. Proper treatment and disposition was given. He was thankful for the ED treatment when he left. There was no injury caused by our treatment. Therefore, he had none of the necessary requirements to initiate a lawsuit. Nevertheless, complaints like these are upsetting and frustrating because they are inaccurate.

Case 10.22 Was it a true miss?

Selbst and Korin present a similar complaint in *Preventing Malpractice Lawsuits in Pediatric Emergency Medicine*.[21] The ED director received a

continued

complaint from the mother of a two-year-old patient. The mother was upset that her child received a misdiagnosis after waiting two hours to be seen. The child was diagnosed with a 'viral infection' and given no medications. The following day, the child's pediatrician found an otitis media and placed the child on antibiotics. Hence, the mother did not feel that she should pay the ED bill and stated that she sent a copy of the complaint to her attorney.

Attorneys are generally not involved in cases of misdiagnoses where no harm was done. This is especially true if their sole purpose is to help a patient avoid paying a medical bill. Although the details of this case are limited, one cannot say with certainty that a misdiagnosis occurred. The exception would be if the ED physician did not look in the child's ears. Viruses can also cause otitis media. What if the clinical findings of otitis media were not yet present during the ED visit? Furthermore, not all cases of otitis media require antibiotics. Therefore, hospital administrators and department directors must substantiate these complaints and stand behind their physicians if they are invalid.

Case 10.23 Valid concerns, wrong approach

The final example of scare tactics in patient complaints also comes from Selbst and Korin's *Preventing Malpractice Lawsuits in Pediatric Emergency Medicine.*[21] The father of a three-year-old boy with leukemia wrote a letter of complaint to the hospital's public relations department. The boy had presented to the ED with fever and neutropenia and was admitted to the hospital. His father was concerned with the amount of time that the boy spent in the ED and the exposure to other sick patients. He had wanted his son to be directly admitted and avoid the ED. The boy's oncologist, however, recommended an evaluation in the ED. The father was an attorney and wrote his letter on his law firm's stationery.

In this case, the child's father had legitimate concerns for his son. Hospitals should have protocols to prevent the spread of communicable diseases to those at risk. Emergency departments should also maintain clean and private rooms for those with increased susceptibility to infections. Elimination of exposure to potential diseases, however, is impossible in the ED setting. We like to think of the ED as the place where we see people when they are not at their best (in fact, some might be at their worse). People do not usually come to the ED when they are healthy, have just bathed, and have put on their Sunday best. They might be living in the woods, working in a ditch, or be covered with stool. Therefore, the father was probably right in wanting his child to be directly admitted. Should his letter of complaint have been addressed to the child's oncologist?

In contrast to the above cases, some complaints have great validity and are handled poorly by physicians because of an 'ego trip.'

Case 10.24 Too many to forgive

Selbst and Korin present a case in *Preventing Malpractice Lawsuits in Pediatric Emergency Medicine* of a 21-year-old woman who presented to an ED after a motor vehicle accident.[22] She was discharged from the ED after the emergency physician had read all of her X-rays as negative. Later that day, the radiologist reviewed the X-rays and saw a 20% pneumothorax, multiple fractured ribs, and fractures of the pelvis and sacrum.

The patient was asked to return to the hospital to receive further care for her injuries. Afterwards, she filed a lawsuit of negligence against the ED physician for $94 in medical expenses. The physician denied any negligence and stated that the patient did not suffer any harm. He also felt that his misinterpretation of the X-rays did not fall below the standard of care for an emergency physician. His opinions, however, were different than that of the courts. They awarded the patient the $94, an additional $2500 for pain and suffering, and additional money from the hospital and insurance company.

The lawsuit, in this case, probably started out as a complaint. The patient was frustrated with receiving a bill (from the physician) for suboptimal medical care. She was most likely seeking compensation for the additional medical visit. The physician was arrogant in not accepting his mistake. Most emergency physicians will occasionally miss an X-ray finding on a visit. Some experienced ED physicians will even miss two X-ray findings on a visit. Missing more than two X-ray findings on a visit, however, is extremely unusual. It is certainly not within the standard of care. Furthermore, pneumothorax, multiple rib fractures, and pelvic fractures are serious findings that must be addressed immediately before a patient is discharged. Therefore, the physician should have been more understanding toward the patient's frustration. This would have led him to write off his bill and avoid fighting an uphill battle.

Worker's compensation issues

Patient's often come to the ED for evaluation of work-related injuries. Their follow-up care is often pre-arranged and delegated to specific physicians. These physicians may not be the same ones that ED physicians would use. The term 'gatekeeper' is often used in the medical care of these patients. After they are treated in the ED, they are often assigned to a particular physician (usually a primary care or urgent care provider). This physician then decides whether specialty referral is needed. This system works extremely well most of the time. There are times, however, where the ED physician's liability is increased.

Case 10.25 Fighting through the gatekeeper

Gardner and Mendelson present a case in *Foresight* where the ED physician is held liable when the patient's follow-up care is delayed.[23] A 42-year-old man accidentally jammed his left hand into the blade of a band saw. His friends applied a tourniquet to his arm and brought him to the ED. The triage nurse removed the tourniquet because the patient's hand was purple. She also ordered an X-ray.

The ED physician examined the patient and noted that there was a laceration that extended from the base of the thumb to the ulnar styloid. He did not see any fractures or foreign bodies. The patient was slightly uncooperative during the examination but seemed to have limited dorsiflexion of the wrist and fingers. The physician then called the orthopedist on call. The orthopedist instructed him to close and splint the wound and have the patient follow up with the occupational medicine clinic the next day.

As instructed, the patient went to the occupational medicine clinic. He complained of numbness in the ring and little fingers. A family practitioner examined him and noted these findings on the physical exam. The patient was then sent home and instructed to take his pain medicines and elevate his arm. Three days later, the patient returned to the clinic. The numbness in his fingers was now accompanied by weakness in his hand. A different physician saw him and did not address these complaints. The patient was given a compressive elastic dressing and told to return in one week.

On the patient's third visit to the clinic, a third clinic physician saw him. This physician ordered an electromyelogram (EMG). This revealed that there was denervation of the ulnar nerve. The patient was referred to a hand surgeon. He underwent a nerve graft of the ulnar nerve, a repair of the radial artery, and a repair of the palmaris longus tendon and flexor digitorum superficialis tendons of the index and middle fingers two weeks later.

After six weeks of physical therapy and rehabilitation, the patient was still left with difficulty of intrinsic hand function and loss of fine motor skills. The patient filed a lawsuit against the ED physician. The other physicians involved in the patient's care were excluded from the lawsuit.

This case was settled against the emergency physician. There was clear medical negligence in this case. However, was the ED physician the only person negligent? Although he did not address the patient's neurovascular injuries, he realized that the patient needed the care of a specialist. He did contact the on-call orthopedist and followed his instructions concerning disposition. The first two clinic physicians, in contrast, failed to recognize and address the patient's injuries appropriately. In addition, are we holding the ED physician responsible for the flaws of the worker's compensation 'gatekeeper' protocol? If we feel that a worker's compensation injury requires the care of a specialist, we should document this in the chart and tell the patient this. We cannot allow the limitations of protocols that do not have medical basis increase our liability.

References

1 Edwards FJ (2002) *The M & M Files: morbidity and mortality rounds in emergency medicine.* Hanley & Belfus Inc., Philadelphia, Pennsylvania, 18–20.
2 Edwards FJ (2002) *The M & M Files: morbidity and mortality rounds in emergency medicine.* Hanley & Belfus Inc., Philadelphia, Pennsylvania, 19–20.
3 Edwards FJ (2002) *The M & M Files: morbidity and mortality rounds in emergency medicine.* Hanley & Belfus Inc., Philadelphia, Pennsylvania, 20.
4 Selbst SM and Korin JB (2003) *Preventing Malpractice Lawsuits in Pediatric Emergency Medicine.* American College of Emergency Physicians, Dallas, Texas, 133.
5 Edwards FJ (2002) *The M & M Files: morbidity and mortality rounds in emergency medicine.* Hanley & Belfus Inc., Philadelphia, Pennsylvania, 94–6.
6 Edwards FJ (2002) *The M & M Files: morbidity and mortality rounds in emergency medicine.* Hanley & Belfus Inc., Philadelphia, Pennsylvania, 100–101.
7 Grassie C, Henry GL and Wagner MJ (2004) Interruptions in patient care. *Foresight: Risk Management for Emergency Physicians.* **59**(February): 2–4.
8 Grassie C, Henry GL and Wagner MJ (2004) Interruptions in patient care. *Foresight: Risk Management for Emergency Physicians.* **59**(February): 2.
9 Wear-Finkle DJ (2000) *Medicolegal Issues in Clinical Practice: a primer for the legally challenged.* Rapid Psychler Press, Port Huron, Michigan, 82.
10 Edwards FJ (2002) *The M & M Files: morbidity and mortality rounds in emergency medicine.* Hanley & Belfus Inc., Philadelphia, Pennsylvania, 180–81.
11 Edwards FJ (2002) *The M & M Files: morbidity and mortality rounds in emergency medicine.* Hanley & Belfus Inc., Philadelphia, Pennsylvania, 201–2.
12 Albert T (2004) Physicians found negligent for not performing CT scan. *American Medical News.* **47**(14): 25.
13 Edwards FJ (2002) *The M & M Files: morbidity and mortality rounds in emergency medicine.* Hanley & Belfus Inc., Philadelphia, Pennsylvania, 211–12.
14 Edwards FJ (2002) *The M & M Files: morbidity and mortality rounds in emergency medicine.* Hanley & Belfus Inc., Philadelphia, Pennsylvania, 220–21.
15 Edwards FJ (2002) *The M & M Files: morbidity and mortality rounds in emergency medicine.* Hanley & Belfus Inc., Philadelphia, Pennsylvania, 222–3.
16 Edwards FJ (2002) *The M & M Files: morbidity and mortality rounds in emergency medicine.* Hanley & Belfus Inc., Philadelphia, Pennsylvania, 222.
17 Selbst SM and Korin JB (2003) *Preventing Malpractice Lawsuits in Pediatric Emergency Medicine.* American College of Emergency Physicians, Dallas, Texas, 94.
18 Selbst SM and Korin JB (2003) *Preventing Malpractice Lawsuits in Pediatric Emergency Medicine.* American College of Emergency Physicians, Dallas, Texas, 96.
19 Edwards FJ (2002) *The M & M Files: morbidity and mortality rounds in emergency medicine.* Hanley & Belfus Inc., Philadelphia, Pennsylvania, 234–6.
20 Selbst SM and Korin JB (2003) *Preventing Malpractice Lawsuits in Pediatric Emergency Medicine.* American College of Emergency Physicians, Dallas, Texas, 126.
21 Selbst SM and Korin JB (2003) *Preventing Malpractice Lawsuits in Pediatric Emergency Medicine.* American College of Emergency Physicians, Dallas, Texas, 153.
22 Selbst SM and Korin JB (2003) *Preventing Malpractice Lawsuits in Pediatric Emergency Medicine.* American College of Emergency Physicians, Dallas, Texas, 156.
23 Gardner AF and Mendelson DJ (2002) Avoidable errors in wound management. *Foresight: Risk Management for Emergency Physicians.* **55**(October): 2–3.

Chapter 11

What to do after you have been sued

- The initial reaction
- Meet your defense attorney
- General rules to follow concerning malpractice litigation
- It is now time for you to do your own investigation
- Make sure that the plaintiff expert witness is competent
- Make sure that your own expert witness is competent
- Write a rebuttal
- Prepare for your deposition and your trial
- Take legal action if warranted
- Decide if the lawsuit is valid

Now that we have spent the previous chapters in this book discussing clinical techniques to avoid legal difficulties, this last chapter is devoted to the actions to take once you are sued. We do not claim to be experts in this scenario because, fortunately, our personal experience has been limited. However, we have read numerous books on this topic and have talked to numerous physicians who have been through the process. From this collection of data, we present the following discussion.

The initial reaction

One of the darkest moments in medicine occurs when a physician receives a letter stating 'intent to initiate litigation.' This is the first notice that the defendant physician usually receives when he is about to be sued. The letter will usually contain the plaintiff attorney's accusations, an affidavit from an expert witness along with his or her curriculum vitae, and questions about the physician from the plaintiff attorney that must be answered in a timely fashion. Do not be surprised to see defamatory and accusatory remarks from the plaintiff attorney concerning your medical care of the patient involved.

Your initial reaction is likely to be a combination of surprise, anger, betrayal, regret, and disparagement. For most of us, this will be a severe blow to our pride of being a good physician. Embarrassment and shame may strike some as they contemplate how to face their families, their staff, their patients, and other physicians. Even for those who might have anticipated the suit, it is still tough for them to avoid the strong emotions that the letter of intent instigates.

The first thing that the physician should do is to put everything in perspective. An 'intent to initiate litigation' letter is an accusation that you have done something wrong. This accusation is someone's opinion and may or may not be correct.

Most of us are not going to remember too many details of the particular patient encounter without reviewing the chart. With the shotgun approach used by plaintiff attorneys, there is a chance that you may not have even been involved in the case (*see* Chapter 8 under 'Frivolous lawsuits'). Refer to **Case 8.16**: in this case we were accused of being an ED physician at a hospital that we did not practice in. Furthermore, we were recently sent an 'intent to initiate litigation' letter on a patient that we never saw. Our name was attached to the suit because the patient had been registered to the ED under our name. Another ED physician, however, treated the patient. Finally, because medical records can be confusing to read and medical signatures difficult to interpret, it is not unusual for the attorney to pinpoint the wrong doctor.

Also realize that getting sued is not uncommon and does not mean that you are an incompetent doctor. We have seen all different kinds of statistics in the literature but we have generally remembered 'the rule of fives.' A doctor averages a lawsuit every five years or after every 5000 patient encounters. That is not a bad average for any profession, much less one that is scrutinized as much as medicine is.

If you do find that you are involved in the case, take comfort in knowing that the statistical odds are still in your favor. The majority of cases will not go to trial, a good number will be eventually dropped, and most trial verdicts are still on the side of the physician.

Meet your defense attorney

After notifying your insurance carrier, it is time to meet your defense attorney. The letter of intent to initiate litigation will contain some questions for you but do not answer these until you have consulted with your attorney. The insurance company will assign you a defense attorney. This does not mean that you are obligated to use this attorney. You have the option of selecting your own attorney (at your expense) and declining the services of the assigned lawyer. You may also have both attorneys work on your case if they are amenable to this.

In your first meeting, make sure that you and your lawyer are both clear with your respective objectives for the case. This will give you a good idea whether you would like to proceed with his services. Is he willing to listen if you feel that he is going in a different direction from you? If not, it is probably in your best interest to find your own attorney.

Remember that the defense attorney is the head coach of your legal defense. You must be comfortable with his personality, experience, enthusiasm, and outlook. He will give you instructions on how to handle each matter that develops during the case. These instructions must be followed without any deviation or you will jeopardize the integrity of your defense. You must also trust that he will select the best expert witness and coordinate a well-organized defense. Any interrogatories from the opposing counsel should be answered with the help of your defense attorney.

Although your lawyer is the head coach, you are the medical coordinator. You must take the time and effort to make sure that your attorney understands the important medical details of the case. Malpractice lawsuits are largely about explaining your case to people with little medical background and being able to convince them that your actions are justified. There is no better person than your attorney on which to start practicing this strategy. Assume that the plaintiff attorney has a fairly broad medical knowledge base about the case (as most will develop before the trial) and even the odds by arming your own lawyer with medical knowledge.

General rules to follow concerning malpractice litigation

These rules are usually discussed during your initial meeting with your defense attorney. Although some of them may seem unfair and unnecessary, you must follow them closely to avoid weakening your case. Do not forget that you are the neophyte at this game and your attorney the seasoned veteran. If you are unclear with any of these rules, 'ask' before you 'do.'

You will be directed to not discuss the case with anyone unless instructed, with the probable exception of your significant other. We found this rule extremely difficult to abide by in our case because of the temptation to discuss your case with colleagues to obtain their support and advice. In addition, if you work in a group practice, your colleagues will likely know that you are involved in a suit and will likely pose questions. This restriction makes it extremely difficult for you to obtain medical opinions to support your case. However, it must be followed to maintain the confidentiality of the parties involved in the suit. In fact, during deposition and at trial, the plaintiff attorney will ask you whether you have discussed the case with any other party besides your attorney. A quote from *Law for Physicians: an overview of medical legal issues* sums up this paragraph: 'it should be assumed by the medical care provider that any information communicated about this incident to anyone other than the attorney (and in rare cases even information communicated to the attorney) will be subject to legal discovery and could be shown to a jury.'[1]

All inquiries that you receive from the plaintiff attorney or the plaintiff must be given to your attorney. Do not try to respond to any before he instructs you to do so. Plaintiff attorneys will sometimes ask inappropriate questions to which you do not have to reply. They often do this with the intent of getting you to volunteer more information. They also like to ask the same question repeatedly in different ways with the hopes that your answers are not consistent. Do not try to outmaneuver their craftiness without the help of your attorney.

You must have an honesty policy with your defense attorney. He cannot help the client who gives false information. This makes both individuals look unorganized and incompetent during deposition and in the courtroom. It also prevents your attorney from making an accurate assessment of the case. A good defense lawyer can assimilate the facts and develop a notion of whether a case is worth taking to trial or is best completed by settlement. The facts, however, must be accurate and true for this notion to be reliable.

You must prove that you are competent to your lawyer. He cannot proudly defend you if he does not believe in you. Before your first meeting, you should have reviewed the details of the case fully and be ready to discuss it. Do not walk into his office and tell him that you do not remember the case and need to review the chart. Your attorney will also give you numerous deadlines to complete. This will include sending him your malpractice insurance papers, your employment contract, your curriculum vitae, your license certificate, etc. It will also include completing the opposing interrogatories by the requested date. These deadlines must be met with promptness and readiness. Lastly, your attorney will ask you many questions concerning the medical facts of the case. It is to your benefit to explain these to him so that he can explain it in layman's terms. Furthermore, you will help your case by researching and copying medical facts, which your attorney can use as exhibits.

Finally, keep in touch with your attorney. Our attorney addressed this issue on our initial meeting. He asked if we would like to be kept abreast of new details as they developed. He said that he had prior physician clients who did not want to be bothered with anything to which they did not have to respond. Do not develop this attitude because learning the legal tactics and process is a significant part of the battle. If your attorney offers this alternative, seize it. If he does not, find one that does.

It is now time for you to do your own investigation

This begins what is called the discovery period in a lawsuit. The discovery period can be further divided into written and verbal periods. The written discovery consists of three forms: requests for admissions, interrogatories, and requests for production of documents.[2] In the requests for admissions, the recipient is given statements that he or she has to admit or deny under oath. Interrogatories are questions concerning the case that must be answered under oath and may be used in trial. Lastly, requests for production of documents enable a party to obtain all of the medical records that may be used in the trial and its proceedings. The verbal discovery period consists of the deposition and that is discussed further later in this chapter.

The written discovery, however, applies to both sides of a malpractice claim. Just because you are the defendant, it does not mean that you should not use these privileges to discover information about your plaintiff. Using **Case 8.15** as an example, we will show how we used these techniques in our own lawsuit. Questions that we used in the requests for admissions to our plaintiff included:

1 Did he ever stop smoking as he was instructed?
2 Did he follow up with the podiatrists who were referred to him?
3 Did he keep all of the appointments that were made for him?
4 Did he take his medications correctly as he was prescribed?

We, of course, had records that we obtained from the requests for production of documents to show that the answers to all of these questions were 'no.' We were able to also discover from obtaining medical records from the podiatrist and the vascular surgeon's offices that the podiatrist had made multiple gross and negligent errors in the patient's treatment, the vascular surgeon was frustrated with the patient's noncompliance, and the podiatrist's disregard for the vascular surgeon's recommendations. Finally, in the interrogatories, we showed that the patient could not give any reasonable explanations as to his noncompliance and negligence of his own medical health.

We mentioned above that the defense attorney is the head coach of the defense team. This does not mean that you should sit on the bench. You are still the starting middle linebacker and must be proactive and a leader in your defense. A suit is a fight against you and you must come out fighting.

After meeting with your attorney, you should obtain all of the medical notes concerning the patient's particular visit. In addition, you should pull all of the visits of that particular patient in your practice to review. Furthermore, your attorney will be able to order from other offices those records to which you would usually not have access.

Go through all of these records with a 'fine tooth comb.' Note trends that may be useful for your defense. For example, did the patient have a habit of noncompliance with medical recommendations (as was the case in our lawsuit)? Did the patient ever give false information to a physician? Did the patient have detrimental social habits such as smoking, illicit drug use, or partaking in promiscuous sexual activities. Has the patient had run-ins with the law?

If you believe that your clinical actions were performed within the standards of care, it is time to prove this to others. Look in current and standard medical texts, updated journals, and protocols from medical organizations for data to support your case. Make copies of this data and give them to your attorney to use as exhibits. Since there is often more than one protocol or standard for the treatment of a certain problem, find as many sources as you possibly can in order to counter the chance that the plaintiff attorney will produce a protocol that is different than yours. Anticipate that the opposing attorney will ask you at some point whether you have treated the particular problem before, how many times you have treated it, and if you have ever had any complications. If your answers to these questions are favorable, document and file your previous cases and be ready to share them.

If you have problems finding the literature to support your actions, recruit your colleagues and mentors. Although we stated above that you are not allowed to discuss the details of the case due to confidentiality issues, this does not prevent you from exchanging some minor details and presenting a 'hypothetical' case to others. After all, this case-based learning is the foundation of medical education. We are fortunate enough to be part of a very colleague-oriented profession. Most physicians will bend over backwards to help another physician.

Make sure that the plaintiff expert witness is competent

Expert witnesses are supposed to be 'expert' in their fields and able to give insight into the standard of care for a particular case. However, we have seen and read through the years the concept of expert witness often being degraded to any physician who the plaintiff attorneys can find to support their opinion and accept their generous allowance. We would also admit that a good number of expert witnesses are legitimate and are concerned with improving the quality of care through their work. We, ourselves, would not have a problem with being an expert witness for a case if we felt that we would render an acceptable recommendation on the standard of care and that there was a clear cut case of medical malpractice. However, we have yet to serve in this capacity.

The first case examples are through our own personal experiences. We mention earlier in Chapter 8 (**Case 8.15**) our lawsuit where the podiatrist served as the expert witness. We believe that there were three legal problems with this podiatrist serving as the expert witness. The first was an issue that concerned our attorney. This was whether a podiatrist's opinion could serve as expert testimony in a case concerning the patient's medical problems (peripheral vascular disease in this case). The second was whether a medical provider who is directly involved in the patient's care could give an impartial expert opinion. With regard to this podiatrist, he had missed the clinical diagnosis of osteomyelitis and disregarded the vascular surgeon's recommendations while performing ill-advised surgery. Therefore, his medical malpractice certainly prevented him from making an impartial opinion. Finally, the podiatrist had a long history of confrontations with the law and this should have prevented him from being a reliable expert witness.

Remember our example in **Case 8.16** of the ED physician from Miami who made a legal affidavit criticizing us for the emergency care of an infant who subsequently died. The child was treated and died at a hospital 100 miles from our hospital. This was four months after we had seen her at our hospital for an unrelated complaint. The expert witness obviously did not review the correct ED chart before making this affidavit. We believe this example should be a model for the incompetence of some expert witnesses. It also demonstrates that some expert witnesses can be extremely careless in their chart review despite receiving generous amounts for this responsibility.

We have seen or read about other expert witnesses that we feel are incapable to render an expert opinion on the standard of care for a case.

Case 11.1 Comparing apples to oranges

A friend of ours who works in the Veterans Administration Hospital (VA) in Florida was in a case where the expert witness was in private practice in Ohio. There are two flaws with this scenario. Anyone who has ever worked in the VA system realizes that medicine is practiced in a slightly different fashion than in private practice. There are no managed health plans; waiting time for certain specialists may be short while other specialists may take longer; formularies are more limited, etc. Therefore, a private practice physician would not work under the same guidelines or standards as a government physician. Lee, in *Legal Concepts and Issues in Emergency Care*, discusses the concept of using the 'failure to provide similarly situated expert' as a defense in medical negligence claims.[3] She writes that 'an expert witness who is "similarly situated" mandates someone currently in the field of practice related to the professional negligence action.'[3]

Secondly, medicine is predominantly a state-regulated activity. Each state has its own process for licensing physicians and its own requirements for continuing education. Each physician is also under the microscope of its own state health agency. Furthermore, with the exception of government physicians, a physician can only practice in a state where he is licensed. Therefore, it makes no sense to us that a physician can vouch for the standard of care in a state where he does not practice. In addition, if you cannot use your medical education to practice medicine in a state in which you are not licensed, why are you able to use your medical education to testify in a court of a state in which you do not hold a license. Indeed, 'according to AMA policy, expert testimony does constitute the practice of medicine.'[4] Therefore, it would be reasonable to expect experts to be licensed in the state that they are testifying in.

Case 11.2 Times change

Another colleague of ours was sued with the help of an expert witness who had not practiced clinical medicine since 1991. Medicine is one of the fastest developing and evolving academic fields. For a plaintiff attorney to extrapolate the experience of a physician from over a decade ago and apply it to a present case is like pulling out a 1969 Volkswagen Beetle and expecting it to have the same features as a 2004 Volkswagen Beetle. This expert witness was not much different from the 'hired gun' physicians that we have read about in medical newsletters. This group of physicians does not practice clinical medicine; rather, they spend the majority or all of their time as expert witnesses. Some even have a posting on the internet to attract plaintiff attorneys. We do not feel that these physicians should be regarded as 'experts' because medicine is an art that you learn as you practice. You do not learn medicine from a book. A great quote from *Law For Physicians: an overview of medical legal issues* supports our beliefs: 'today's accepted standard of care can become tomorrow's archaic quackery a lot faster than used to be the case.'[5]

There are a few other issues to make sure that you check your expert witness. Research the National Practitioner Data Bank to see if he or she has ever been sued. If they have been sued more than the national average, then they can be accused of being 'the pot calling the kettle black.' Is the physician board-certified in their specialty? Although it is controversial whether board certification equates to a better clinician, it is the standard criterion by which most people judge a physician's qualification. Does the physician ever testify for the defense or is he strictly a plaintiff witness? A bipartisan witness is more likely to provide an impartial opinion.

Case 11.3 They saw right through him

Tanya Albert writes about a case in *American Medical News* in which the plaintiff's expert witness took an unusual step to try to convince the jury that he was competent.[6] In this case, a gynecologist was on trial for a failed tubal ligation. The plaintiff's expert was a board-certified obstetrics-gynecology physician who had reviewed the initial operative report, the operative report from the resterilization, and the pathology report. When he was called to the stand, he claimed that 'the procedure was inappropriately performed and did not meet the standard of care.'[7] His arguments were that the tube did not have adequate time after surgery to recanalize and that the ring was not applied correctly around the fallopian tube. He could not produce, however, any studies to support his notion of the time frame that it would take for a tube to recanalize. When he was asked to comment on the pathology report, which stated that the ring was in the correct location and that the tube had recanalized, the physician stated: 'I accept [the pathologist's] report; I don't accept her conclusion.'[7]

continued

The defense also discovered that the physician had served as an expert witness 23 times in the past 15 years and had testified in 18 different states. When he was asked of the last time that he had performed a tubal ligation, he replied that he had completed one that morning. It was later brought out during the trial that the physician had previously not done a tubal ligation in 10 years before the one in the morning. The jurors were not impressed with this witness because he was not willing to accept any other explanation for the outcome than his own, despite reports suggesting otherwise. They also felt that he had purposely scheduled the tubal ligation that morning to impress them. Lastly, he came unprepared and without any supporting documents to defend his beliefs. Please see the next section for the actions of the defendant expert witness in this case.

Case 11.4 A change of heart

In our final example from Ronald Schwarz in *Medical Economics*, the plaintiff's expert witness in this case was also not credible.[8] After having lumbar spinal surgery, a 70-year-old man developed a post-operative ileus. Dr Schwarz, a gastroenterologist, was consulted to evaluate and treat this problem. He ordered serum electrolytes and stopped the patient's narcotics.

The physician's partner, another gastroenterologist, covered for him over the weekend. During this time, the second physician had corrected the patient's electrolyte imbalance. When the first physician returned on Monday, the patient had developed worsening hemodynamic status as evidenced by clinical fluid overload and fluctuating blood pressure. Later that evening, the patient went into cardiopulmonary arrest. He vomited and aspirated during the arrest but was able to be resuscitated at the expense of severe neurologic damage. He was taken off life support two days later.

Approximately two years later, the patient's family filed a lawsuit against the hospital, the two cardiologists, the gastroenterologist, and his partner. The plaintiff had the choice of two stands to take, that of sudden cardiac death or that of aspiration. They chose to pursue that of aspiration and faulted the gastroenterologists for not ordering the placement of a nasogastric suctioning tube. This choice led to the cardiologists being dropped from the case and the hospital decided to settle. Therefore, the case was left against the two gastroenterologists.

The gastroenterologists were distraught because there had been clues that the patient might have died from a cardiac cause. The patient's blood pressure was 76/40 mm/Hg (about half of what it had been) one hour before his arrest. He was alert and oriented prior to his arrest, which goes against aspiration. In addition, the autopsy report determined that the cause of death was an arrhythmia, with only minimal changes of aspiration pneumonia (which the patient had during the arrest). Even with these facts

continued

as evidence, the case proceeded to trial with the accusation that the patient died from aspiration.

At trial, there was a three-hour videotape testimony from the plaintiff expert witness. He was a cardiologist who was also used as the expert witness against the two defendant cardiologists before they were dropped from the case. He now argued that he did not find any fault with the care of the cardiologists. He stated that the patient did not have a history of heart problems and could not have experienced an arrhythmia. In light of the autopsy findings, this statement was analogous to a criminal denying a crime where his fingerprints are collected and identified. This witness should also have been asked to explain the pre-arrest hypotension, the clinical fluid overload, and the fluctuating blood pressure. Finally, it would have been helpful for the jury to know the last time and the number of times that this cardiologist had treated a postoperative ileus. If the answer is a long time ago and a few times, respectively, then his three hours of testimony should be taken in the context of his inexperience. Incidentally, the jury found in favor of the gastroenterologists in this case.

Make sure that your own expert witness is competent

Most defendant attorneys will ask you to choose an expert witness. This will not always be the case, however, because we surmise that defendant attorneys have a pool of 'hired guns' themselves. It would be nice to have an active role in picking your expert witness because you can avoid some of the pitfalls stated above. Ideally, you want to pick someone with an outstanding medical and personal background. They should also be practicing clinically in your state and in a practice similar to yours. Some defense lawyers will also prefer that the physician be someone that you do not know personally so that they can give an impartial opinion.

By selecting an expert witness who has few or no flaws, you create certain advantages for your case. The opposing attorney will have less chance of attack on the expert witness's credentials. Your defense will become more credible with the opinions of a respected expert. Finally, you and your lawyer can attack the credentials of the plaintiff's expert witness if the court allows such activity.

With regard to **Case 11.3**, the defendant expert witness in this case served as a good model to seek for your own case.[7] He was a board-certified obstetrics-gynecology physician from the same area as the trial. His experience was extensive and current in the area for which he was testifying. He had performed over 100 tubal ligations and was currently averaging two or three per year. In 20-plus years of involvement in almost 50 malpractice cases, his participation had been 40% of the time for the plaintiffs and 60% of the time for the defendants.

He reviewed the same reports as the plaintiff's expert witness and reiterated that the reports supported the notion that the standard of care was met. He acknowledged that tubal ligation procedures could be performed incorrectly but that there was nothing in the reports to suggest that this was the case. Furthermore, he stated that recanalization can occur in six months. The jury found this expert witness more comforting to believe than the plaintiff's witness and, subsequently, returned a verdict in favor of the defense.

The final point is to consider an expert witness from the case. A physician who had first-hand involvement with treating the patient lends credibility. This person may be extremely helpful to a defense and counter the arguments of the plaintiff's expert witness. Most people will agree that there are usually intangibles to a case that only an insider could comment on. Hence, the plaintiff expert witness would not have this advantage unless he or she was involved in the patient's care.

In **Case 8.15**, the plaintiff received treatment from a vascular surgeon. The surgeon stated repeatedly in his progress notes that he was frustrated with the patient's unwillingness to stop smoking. He was also displeased with the patient's many missed appointments. He criticized the patient as 'doctor shopping' when the patient sought the care of a second vascular surgeon. The biggest intangible that we believed he could have brought to the case was his criticism of the podiatrist's decision to perform surgery on the plaintiff. He was openly critical of this in his progress notes.

In our discussions with our defense attorney, we were prepared to ask the surgeon to testify. We felt strongly that his comments would be damaging to the plaintiff's case. More importantly, we were confident that the comments of the plaintiff expert witness (the podiatrist) would be negated by the surgeon's testimony. Finally, in our review of all of the patient's records, we discovered that many of the other physicians who took care of the patient acknowledged the same issues with him as we had. Therefore, we could have also obtained their testimony.

Write a rebuttal

As discussed above, the letter of intent to initiate litigation will contain harsh and defaming language criticizing your treatment of the patient. This criticism will come from the plaintiff attorney and his expert witness. In many situations, you will feel that the content of this letter is inaccurate and/or false. For these situations, it is time to reply to their remarks.

Take our own case example, **Case 8.15**. When we first read the opinion of the expert witness, he stated that our care of the patient was inadequate and below the standard of care. Later, when our attorney was able to obtain the other medical records, the details of the case became more evident. With this new information, we were able to determine the true events that took place and realized that the statements in the affidavit were not correct.

The podiatrist had inappropriately missed the diagnosis of osteomyelitis and had twice performed ill-advised surgery on the patient. These two factors were direct contributors towards the patient's poor outcome. Consequently, we were able to determine that the podiatrist was the one that was guilty of medical malpractice. He then volunteered to serve as the expert witness as a cover-up. We wrote a formal 20-page rebuttal consisting of over 10 medical references supporting our claim of the podiatrist's errors. We included exhibits from the podiatrist's notes demonstrating how he documented findings consistent with osteomyelitis but did not initiate appropriate therapy. We also showed that the vascular surgeon's notes documented his disapproval of the podiatrist's actions.

This rebuttal was given to our attorney as exhibits for use during the deposition and/or trial. It gave him the impression that our case was extremely defendable. We believe that it was one of the major factors that led to the case being dropped.

A final comment on rebuttals is to resist your temptation to reveal them. In our case, once we read the podiatrist's notes and realized that he was at fault, we wanted to call the plaintiff attorney immediately. We believed that it would embarrass him and his expert witness. This is not an intelligent strategy, however, for it may give the plaintiff attorney a chance to come up with another frivolous complaint or change his focus. Save the rebuttal for the depositions or the trial, when the discussions are under oath and recorded. You will catch them by surprise and unprepared to respond.

Prepare for your deposition and your trial

We will not discuss this section in too much detail because our experience with it has been extremely limited. Most of our discussion is based on our reading. The most important things to keep in mind are to be prepared, be professional, and listen to your attorney. As we will elaborate, these three conditions are sometimes difficult to fulfill in a deposition or a trial.

It is tough to keep the details of the case in your head vividly a couple of years later when your deposition or your trial arises. You must, however, refresh yourself on the case when the time approaches so that you have most of the details in memory and not have to refer to the medical records. This is no easy task because most lawsuits will consist of numerous medical records from multiple providers. However, being familiar with the events that occurred with the patient will not only assist you with your responses to the plaintiff attorney's questions, but it will also let everyone know that you cared about the case and did your homework. Meet with your attorney prior to either event to stage a mock run and discuss the anticipated questions. An experienced defense attorney can just about tell you the exact type of questions that the opposing counsel will bring up.

Although your clinical ability is being questioned during a deposition or a trial, maintaining professionalism is still a top priority. Dress and groom yourself appropriately and conservatively. We read about an elderly Texas physician who went to his trial in boots and a cowboy hat. We do not need to mention the outcome of his trial. The opposing counsel will do his best with different tactics to try to rattle you. It is his trial run for the strategy that he will use in court. You will frustrate them the most if you can maintain your composure through anything that he may throw at you. This is much easier said than done.

During our deposition, the plaintiff attorney did arouse our anger with a couple of statements of accusation. Our attorney, however, was right next to us and was quick at defusing our anger. Finally, it is unnecessary to say that you should address everyone appropriately, use language that is not offensive, and express your regrets for the patient's unfortunate outcome. One final strategy that we used was that we offered to help the plaintiff attorney. Since depositions and trials are publicly recorded events, this gesture of assistance gives the impression that you are confident with your case and have nothing to fear. We told the opposing counsel that we would send him some medical records that he was missing during our deposition.

In contrast, the patient that sued us was anything but professional. He showed up to the deposition and did not appear to be interested in the proceedings. He was rude and used profanity during his deposition. It is amazing that a plaintiff attorney had the courage to accept him as a client. This was the other major factor that led to the case being dropped.

It is extremely important, at these events, to listen to your attorney. Again, the plaintiff attorney will try to instigate and disrupt your composure in the hope that you will burst into outrage or state damaging comments to your case. Your defense attorney will know when this is about to happen and will provide you with cues (visual, auditory, etc.). Be on the alert for these cues. Do not answer a question hastily or reflexively. There is no time limit to a question. A deposition or a trial is not a race. It is more a test of wills. There will be times when you feel that you need to offer information that is not requested (believing that it will help your case). Resist this temptation unless your attorney approves of it. Nothing excites a plaintiff attorney more than a runaway mouth. Remember that one of the goals of the attorney during the deposition is to 'pin down the witness's testimony to keep it from changing.'[9]

Take legal action if warranted

In **Case 8.15**, we could have filed a complaint of medical liability against the podiatrist. Horn, Caldwell, and Osborn discuss in *Law For Physicians: an overview of medical legal issues* that complaints of medical liability can be made as cross-complaints against other defendants or as a third-party complaint against an as yet unnamed party.[10] We believed that the podiatrist in our case was negligent in missing the diagnosis of osteomyelitis and subsequent inappropriate treatment of the patient. He was also negligent in performing an amputation of the patient's toe when a vascular surgeon had advised against it. If our case had gone to trial, we are confident that the podiatrist would have been found liable for the patient's injuries.

Horn, Caldwell, and Osborn also stress that there are other legal actions that the defense should consider.[11] If the defense feels that the lawsuit is in violation of the statute of limitations or the statute of repose, then it can file a motion to dismiss. The statute of limitations varies from state to state but is usually within two to four years. The clock does not start ticking, however, until the alleged harm or injury has manifested.[12] In some cases, such as pediatric cases, the clock is on hold until the patient reaches the adult age of 18. Statutes of repose, in contrast, are used by some states, and are based on time frames that begin from the time of treatment and not from the time of injury.

Case 11.5 Time is up

Starr presents a case, in *Cortlandt Forum*, where a physician benefited from the statute of limitations.[13] A 42-year-old woman had a routine screening Pap smear. An employee of the laboratory (owned by a pathologist) interpreted the smear as 'within normal limits' and reported this result to her gynecologist. The patient saw her gynecologist three years later for

continued

vaginal bleeding. Evaluation revealed that the patient had Stage 3 cervical carcinoma. She died 10 months later.

The patient's husband did not initially want to file a lawsuit against the laboratory. The financial hardships of raising six children by himself caused him to change his mind. He met with a plaintiff attorney four years after the alleged incorrect Pap smear reading. The attorney filed and received a 90-day extension on the statute of limitations. One year after the state's mandatory waiting period expired, the attorney filed the necessary paperwork to initiate the suit.

When the pathologist received the lawsuit papers against the laboratory, he contacted a defense attorney. The defense petitioned to have the case dismissed because the statute of limitations in the state of the claim was four years. The plaintiff attorney, however, argued that this statute of limitations should be extended if 'fraud, concealment, or intentional misrepresentation of fact prevented discovery of the injury.'[14] His contention was that the laboratory's failure to inform the patient of her abnormal Pap smear, whether this failure was intentional or not, represented concealment to the plaintiffs. The defense countered that they were unaware that the Pap smear was abnormal and that there was no intentional concealment. The verdict was in favor of the defense.

During the investigation, it was discovered that the technician was unsure of the appearance of the cells on the Pap smear. He did not, however, present the slide to a senior technician or a pathologist to review. Therefore, the plaintiff probably had enough evidence to win this case. His default was that he waited too long to file the lawsuit.

Another strategy that the defendant physician can use is a stand of independent intervening negligence of some other person and contributory or comparative negligence by the plaintiff.[11] The concept of independent intervening negligence of some other person is similar to the third-party complaint against an as yet unnamed party discussed earlier in this section. In our example **Case 8.15**, the podiatrist's negligence would be a perfect example of intervening negligence.

The argument of contributory or comparative negligence by the plaintiff is one that is frequently used by physicians and defense attorneys. Patients who are non-compliant, neglectful of their own health, or engage in high-risk activities are good examples of plaintiff negligence. In **Case 8.15**, we could probably write a short book on how negligent our patient was in his health and in his noncompliance with medical instructions. We discussed in Chapter 8 under the heading 'New tactics for malpractice lawsuits by attorneys' that a number of jury verdicts now are broken down into percentages of fault. The physician has to show that the plaintiff was at greater than 50% at fault in order to avoid a payment to him or her. Therefore, it is to the physician's benefit to discover every potential error the patient made with his or her healthcare.

Decide if the lawsuit is valid

This final section is one of the difficult ones for a physician to write. We are all frustrated with the medical liability crisis and all claim that there are too many frivolous lawsuits. However, we can see from this book that bad medicine and unfortunate outcomes exist in the practice of medicine. Regardless of the education and the training, there will always be individuals who are lazy and careless. In addition, there are always situations that are no-win situations for everyone involved.

As a professional, it is our duty to decide for ourselves when a preventable mistake or error has occurred. It is our opinion that these cases should be settled as quickly as possible. It not only saves the cost of prolonged litigation efforts on both parties, it also is a lot less stressful for both sides involved. You will also have more to lose professionally if you decide to fight a case that you have a very low chance of winning. Your errors and unwillingness to accept them will be revealed to a greater number of individuals. It is better to accept this event as one that occurred when you were not at your best and let it serve as a learning issue for the future. Remember that our goal is to not fight every lawsuit, because sometimes we need to be faulted and sometimes patients need to be compensated. Our goal, rather, is to avoid practicing careless and substandard medicine and to fight the frivolous lawsuits and the incompetent expert witnesses.

References

1   Horn C, Caldwell DH and Osborn DC (2000) *Law For Physicians: an overview of medical legal issues*. American Medical Association, Chicago, Illinois, 51.
2   Horn C, Caldwell DH and Osborn DC (2000) *Law For Physicians: an overview of medical legal issues*. American Medical Association, Chicago, Illinois, 83.
3   Lee NG (2001) *Legal Concepts and Issues in Emergency Care*. WB Saunders Company, Philadelphia, Pennsylvania, 218.
4   Rice B (2004) Malpractice: Who should judge the experts? *Medical Economics.* **81**(20): 28.
5   Horn C, Caldwell DH and Osborn DC (2000) *Law For Physicians: an overview of medical legal issues*. American Medical Association, Chicago, Illinois, 43.
6   Albert T (2004) Dr Diakos on trial. *American Medical News.* **47**(12): 12–14.
7   Albert T (2004) Dr Diakos on trial. *American Medical News.* **47**(12): 13.
8   Schwarz RP (2004) The separate worlds of the physician-defendant. *Medical Economics.* **81**(7): 68–72.
9   Horn C, Caldwell DH and Osborn DC (2000) *Law For Physicians: an overview of medical legal issues*. American Medical Association, Chicago, Illinois, 85.
10 Horn C, Caldwell DH and Osborn DC (2000) *Law For Physicians: an overview of medical legal issues*. American Medical Association, Chicago, Illinois, 73.
11 Horn C, Caldwell DH and Osborn DC (2000) *Law For Physicians: an overview of medical legal issues*. American Medical Association, Chicago, Illinois, 76.
12 Horn C, Caldwell DH and Osborn DC (2000) *Law For Physicians: an overview of medical legal issues*. American Medical Association, Chicago, Illinois, 74.
13 Starr DS (2004) In this misread Pap smear case, timing is everything. *Cortlandt Forum.* **17**(2): 82–3.
14 Starr DS (2004) In this misread Pap smear case, timing is everything. *Cortlandt Forum.* **17**(2): 83.

Index